CW01238289

Truck It!

BOBBY BOLTON

Truck It!

The Drive Around the World
That Saved My Life

MACMILLAN

First published 2025 by Macmillan
an imprint of Pan Macmillan
The Smithson, 6 Briset Street, London EC1M 5NR
EU representative: Macmillan Publishers Ireland Ltd, 1st Floor,
The Liffey Trust Centre, 117–126 Sheriff Street Upper,
Dublin 1 D01 YC43
Associated companies throughout the world

ISBN 978-1-0350-7447-1 HB

Copyright © Bobby Bolton 2025

The right of Bobby Bolton to be identified as the
author of this work has been asserted in accordance
with the Copyright, Designs and Patents Act 1988.

All rights reserved. No part of this publication may be reproduced,
stored in a retrieval system, or transmitted, in any form, or by any means
(including, without limitation, electronic, mechanical, photocopying, recording or otherwise)
without the prior written permission of the publisher.

Pan Macmillan does not have any control over, or any responsibility for,
any author or third-party websites (including, without limitation, URLs,
emails and QR codes) referred to in or on this book.

1 3 5 7 9 8 6 4 2

A CIP catalogue record for this book is available from the British Library.

Map artwork by Atomic Squib

Typeset in Fairfield LT Std by Palimpsest Book Production Ltd, Falkirk, Stirlingshire
Printed and bound in the UK using 100% Renewable Electricity by CPI Group (UK) Ltd

MIX
Paper | Supporting
responsible forestry
FSC® C116313

This book is sold subject to the condition that it shall not, by way of
trade or otherwise, be lent, hired out, or otherwise circulated without
the publisher's prior consent in any form of binding or cover other than
that in which it is published and without a similar condition including this
condition being imposed on the subsequent purchaser.
The publisher does not authorize the use or reproduction of any part of this book in any
manner for the purpose of training artificial intelligence technologies or systems. The publisher
expressly reserves this book from the Text and Data Mining exception in accordance with
Article 4(3) of the European Union Digital Single Market Directive 2019/790.

Visit **www.panmacmillan.com** to read more about all
our books and to buy them.

I'd like to dedicate this book to Paula and Eagle, who are a 'forever nomadic' couple we met on the road on the shores of Issyk-Kul in Kyrgyzstan.

They epitomize the soul of those who were brought up in 'normal' European life, and left it all behind to explore the world, and never looked back. For them, and others, there is no social media, no book deal, no big following. But that makes their stories and their journey even more captivating.

They, and other global adventurers, continue to inspire *us* to chase our dreams.

So, I hope this book will inspire *you* to take your own leap of faith and explore this little planet we call home.

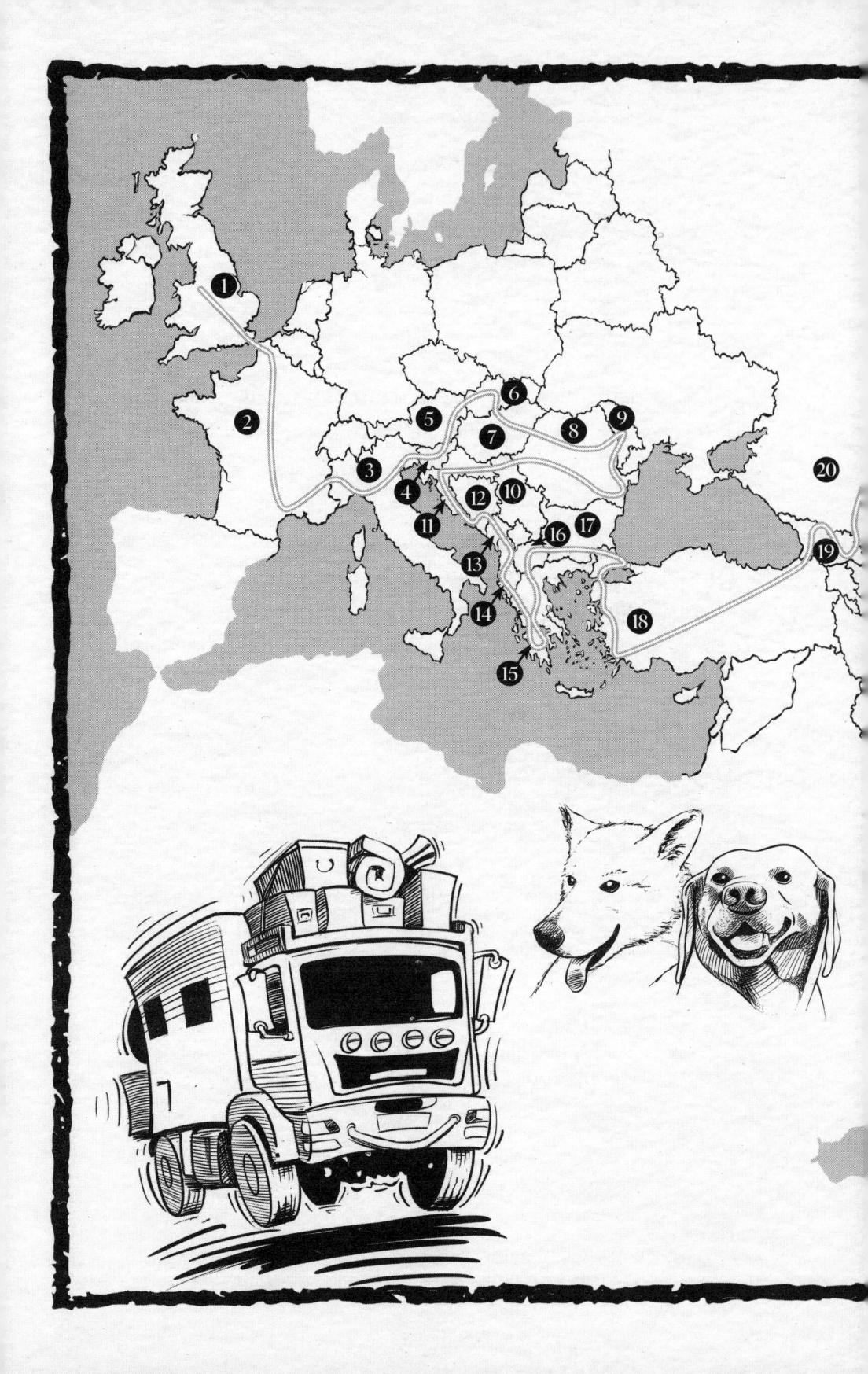

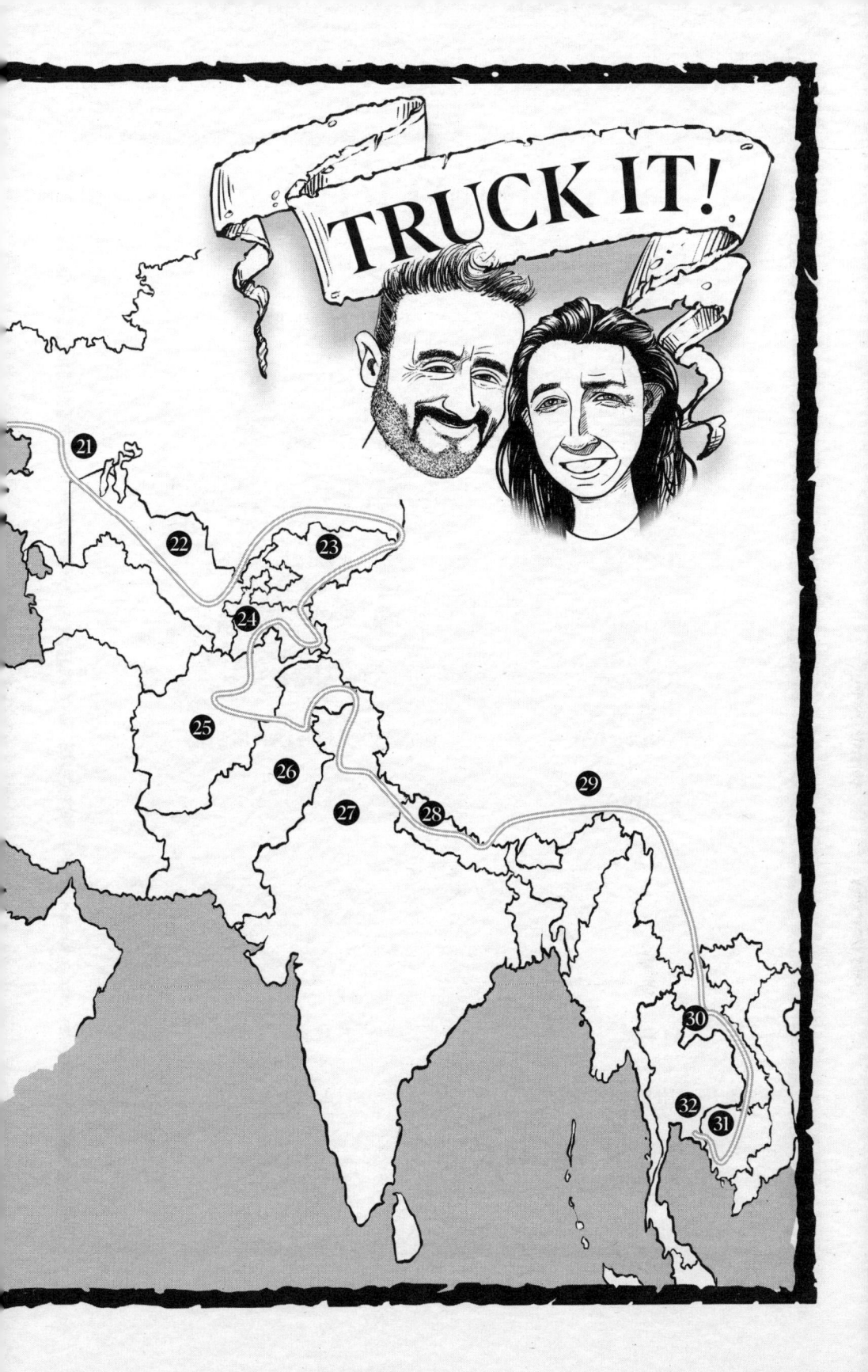

TRUCK IT!

COUNTRIES

1 UNITED KINGDOM

2 FRANCE

3 ITALY

4 SLOVENIA

5 AUSTRIA

6 SLOVAKIA

7 HUNGARY

8 ROMANIA

9 MOLDOVA

10 SERBIA

11 CROATIA

12 BOSNIA

13 MONTENEGRO

14 ALBANIA

15 GREECE

16 NORTH MACEDONIA

17 BULGARIA

18 TURKEY

19 GEORGIA

20 RUSSIA

21 KAZAKHSTAN

22 UZBEKISTAN

23 KYRGYZSTAN

24 TAJIKISTAN

25 AFGHANISTAN

26 PAKISTAN

27 INDIA

28 NEPAL

29 CHINA

30 LAOS

31 CAMBODIA

32 THAILAND

'Don't let who you are today, stop you from being who you could be tomorrow'

Bobby Bolton, 2023

Contents

Introduction: The End of the Beginning   1

1. Why Not?   5
2. Bon Voyage   17
3. Boy Meets Girl   27
4. The Italian Job   38
5. What's French for 'Detour'?   51
6. Slovenia, I Hardly Knew Her?   60
7. Moldova the Top   68
8. Romanic   84
9. Resolutions in Romania   95
10. Montenegro M G   104
11. Istanbullish   112
12. Ups and Downs   126
13. Snow Problem   139
14. Russian Rushing   153

15.	Stanning the Stans	164
16.	Buzzing in Kyrgyzstan	173
17.	Horsing Around in Kyrgyzstan	181
18.	Mars Landing, Tajikistan	194
19.	The Long Road to Kabul	210
20.	Dinner with the Taliban	231
21.	A Relaxing Drive Through Pakistan	246
22.	The Banks of the Ganges	263
23.	Everest and Other Adventures	273
24.	Tibetter or Worse	279
25.	Laos	288

Epilogue   299
Acknowledgements   305

Introduction
The End of the Beginning

'Where are you from?!'
   'Why are you here?!'
   'Is this your wife?!'
   'Are you a spy?!'
   The questions were relentless.
   We were surrounded by thirty or more Taliban soldiers with guns as we sat on a rickety old bench blinking in the bright floodlights. Surreally, there was a volleyball court in the field in front of us. I tried to answer but immediately there was another question fired from a silhouette looming over us. By my side was Marie, the amazing French woman who had put her life on hold to come with me on this trip. I tried to catch her eye, but the headscarf made it hard to see her facial expression. I sat slightly forward on the bench, both hands on one leg, and looked back up at the crowd with my head held high in an attempt to give the impression that I wasn't panicking as I answered: 'England. Travelling. Yes. No.'

Every time I answered, one guy, who had especially wild eyes lined with thick black kohl, kept twisting his head to the side like a dog in a way that sent shivers down my spine. At one point he came striding over and put one foot on the bench, leaning down to peer at me. I tried to telepathically send Marie the message that she should look away, absolutely sure he was going to go at me with a knife.

Drowning out the fear, there was guilt. That I had dragged Marie and the dogs along with me on this adventure. I mean, who does this? Who gives up everything – their job, their house and belongings, their entire life – to drive from Wigan to Australia? Of course something like this was going to happen. How could I be so stupid?! We had been on a journey of 10,0000 miles and at that moment, I didn't think we were going to make it a step further. *This is why normal blokes from Wigan don't do this sort of thing, Bobby!*

I thought back to almost three years before, when my fiancée had called off our engagement after eleven years together, and the construction business I'd sunk my life into had hit the rocks.

While in the depths of those lonely moments that came after the heartbreak, I barely had enough money to buy a coffee on the way in to work and was living in a mouldy caravan. It was like a big, hard, slow kick in the bollocks of my soul.

But, much like a kick to the actual bollocks, it forced me to stop.

I realized that I was so caught up in the rat race that I had lost my way. I had lost who I really was. Who I *wanted* to be.

Truck It!

My dreams of a life of adventure had fallen by the wayside, replaced with the burden of responsibility. A job. A flat. Council tax. The property ladder. The boiler. All this bloody stuff that is part of life. Of growing up. It had never felt like the right time, but I realized that there's never a right time. Because change is always scary. So we just let ourselves remain stuck.

My trip was about unsticking myself. Reminding myself that life is about the journey, not the destination.

However, at this exact moment, I realized there wasn't much point in discovering the meaning of my life if I lost my *actual* life. More importantly, I thought of Marie, how she'd only known me for two weeks before joining me on our trip to see the world. How passionate and funny and beautiful she was. She didn't sign up for this. I thought of my dog Red, my best friend in the whole world, and Rubia. We had left them in the truck with the air conditioning on, but in about eight hours the battery would run out. Then what? They didn't deserve any of this.

I thought of my family and friends at home, waking up to the news. I thought of what people would say. *Stupid tourists getting themselves killed. So needless. So stupid. So naive. What a waste.*

A big guy who towered over the others pushed his way towards us.

'You come now,' he shouted.

Bobby, how the bloody hell did you end up here?

1

Why Not?

'Screw it. I'm driving to Australia.' Cue amounts of laughter normally reserved for someone's trousers falling down.

'Hang on, it was Mongolia a minute ago!' laughed one of my mates. He had a point. About two hours (and five pints) previously, we had been stood outside the pub on a crisp wintery afternoon when a beat-up old Land Rover Defender had pulled up and an outdoorsy couple sprung out, with wild, unkempt hair, muddy boots and fiery looks of adventure in their eyes. There was a sticker on the door that read 'Family Expedition' and the Landy was full of snorkels, shovels and spotlights. It was then I'd decided that I was going to buy a Land Rover and drive to Mongolia. There was something in that couple's eyes that seemed so alive. And I just felt so . . . lost.

Bobby Bolton

Whatever they had, I wanted it.

The previous year had been the hardest of my life. I had lost, in quick succession, my fiancée, who I'd been with for eleven years, and my flat, and my business was hanging by a thread. I had also lost my passion for playing rugby (and anyone who knows me knows what a big deal this is). I was, at that point, living in an ancient mouldy caravan on a farm with no running water, electricity or toilet. At one point, my neighbours, a group of travellers, 'accidentally' shot at my dog, Red, and me, then threatened to smash my head in if I told anyone. I would sit in that caravan, sipping on discounted Tesco pea and ham soup, and replay the moment when my fiancée had turned to me and said we were 'growing apart'. That was the starting pistol for several months of soul-sapping misery that completely crushed my confidence.

Up until that point, life had been great. My fiancée and I had met when we were both at university. We moved south because that suited her career, bought a flat and got a Labrador puppy: Red. After a couple of years, I left my engineering job and even though I'd never picked up much other than a sweeping brush and a clipboard on a building site, I began to pursue the life of a self-employed builder. We bought an old van and I converted it into a camper.

Life was frantic and hard work, but it was utterly fantastic. In my twenties, I had enough motivation to fuel a power station and the work ethic to match. Four years in, the business was turning over a few million a year, I had built the in-house team up to nineteen, and on our busiest day had forty-five men and women working on our building sites. We even won an award, and to celebrate I bought a Range Rover with *said in hushed ashamed tones* white leather seats, formerly owned by a professional footballer. (I know, I know . . .) I felt like I'd earned it, having not paid myself one penny in the first two years of the business. We were embarking on one of the biggest construction projects we'd ever worked on and had managed to borrow enough money to buy an old barn in London and convert it into a luxury house. I remember my eyes filling with tears of pride as I walked into the barn. I was twenty-nine; I had a loyal and hardworking team surrounding me doing good work I believed in and a fiancée I loved.

But the moment of success was to be short-lived.

Two months after we'd put the first spade in the ground on our big conversion job, my fiancée first told me we had grown apart. At exactly the moment I needed to focus on salvaging my relationship, the business hit massive turbulence. First the housing market declined, then two key staff members had to take time off because of family emergencies. We were defrauded, then a client refused to pay us the full amount they owed. Four sales fell through. Then our two flagship developments both suffered illegal activity that tanked their potential value. I had taken on £2 million in debt to buy and convert the barn and was massively overleveraged. I'd had to throw in every single penny I personally had to plug any holes created by the rise in material prices which followed Brexit, the pandemic and the war in Ukraine.

I desperately tried to keep things going. I spent a quarter of my time in tears, half of my time attempting to rescue the relationship, and the final quarter badly managing the business. My motivation was destroyed.

Bobby Bolton

The day my relationship finally ended, I had gone to enquire about a toupee . . . Losing my hair at a young age had always been a bugbear. Conversely, it was great for business as it made me look a lot older. But now, with my confidence on the rocks, it was time to see what options there were. I was fussed over by four beautiful, kind and genuinely caring women who muttered reassuringly about how great it looked. And it was there I looked myself in the mirror and said for the first time: *Bobby, what the hell are you doing here?*

I hardly recognized myself. My shoulders drooped, my back was bent and the bags under my eyes were a permanent feature. I'd lost an awful lot of weight. I had become a shadow of my former self. That night we officially called it off and I packed my bags and marched out the door of the flat with Red in tow and drove off in the campervan. My now ex-fiancée lent me enough money to buy a ten-year-old Elddis caravan.

I spent my thirtieth birthday in that caravan parked on a derelict farm in Hertfordshire.

It was a lonely Sunday, with Henry, a real dear friend, making a big detour on his way home from a weekend away to share a quick barbecue with me to cheer me up.

The caravan had no running water or electricity and I quickly found out that it leaked and had mould growing behind the seats. I cleared an abandoned barn and managed to squeeze the old girl underneath to keep the worst of the rain off, not before being attacked and swarmed by ground-nesting hornets for the first three days. Poor Red took the brunt of the stings, including one particularly nasty one on the todger. For the first few weeks, he flat-out refused to come in unless he was carried.

Electricity came from a petrol generator, and we got our water from an outside tap by a commercial welder's business round the corner. So each night I would wander round with my bucket to fill up enough to wash the dishes and brush my teeth, before stripping off in front of the CCTV cameras to have an ice-cold soapy shower, bending the tap to forty-five degrees to spray upwards. I didn't have the confidence to socialize. I was completely broke, and the guy who used to jump out of bed early every morning to attack the day was gone. My parents had separated when I was a teenager and I'd grown up with them living apart, but I had always been really close to both of them. In classic northern dad style, he hoped this period of my life would be character-building, but Mum was worried sick.

One lonely night sat under blankets in my caravan, using Red as a furry hot-water bottle, I rang my dad and said, 'I can't believe it, Dad. I can't believe how quick it's all fallen apart.' I will never forget his reply:

'Just as quick as it's all fallen apart, it could all fall back into place.'

In order to get our barn conversion project finished and ready to sell, I slept in the campervan outside the site for the final month. I worked throughout the day and night, doing whatever I could to get it over the line. On one fateful day, I drove to the petrol station to get a coffee and didn't even have enough money for that. The available funds in my bank accounts added up to less than 70p. I rooted around in the glove box, blowing off sand and mud to scavenge enough coppers before arriving and putting on a brave face.

A few painful months later, while potential buyers came and went, I drove the 300 miles back north to Wigan to spend a weekend with my friends and family. And that was when I saw the Land Rover with the 'Family Expedition' bumper sticker. That night in the pub, they thought it was just the beer talking.

'Australia is an island, Bobby mate. And it's ten thousand miles away,' one said.

I looked at the (admittedly blurry) map on my phone and traced a line with my finger.

'Well, feck it,' I said in response. 'I don't care. I'm going for it! We only have one life and I want to go and live mine. I'm sick of feeling sorry for myself. Laugh all you want, but I'm going to make this happen.'

The seed had been planted.

Now I just needed to crack on with it.

I began by gifting the construction business to my business partner, closing the offices and liquidating everything I could at a massive loss. It was all bearable, though, because I'd now found a new purpose. A few weeks into the cull, I stumbled upon a fifteen-year-old four-wheel-drive truck, formerly used on muddy construction sites around the country, which had been sat for sale for two years. It was six metres long, two and a half metres wide and weighed six and a half tonnes. It was love at first sight. I knew this was going to be my ticket to freedom.

I had always been interested in trucks, and my grandad had me driving and changing gears as soon as I could reach the pedals. I learnt to drive in a long-wheelbase, single-cab Series 3 Land Rover with a snapped chassis and an engine that took half an hour to start.

Growing up, I'd driven a variety of knackered dumpers, mini diggers and quads on the land behind ours and our grandad's house in the wilds of rural Wigan.

I came from a long line of tinkerers. Both my grandad and dad were constantly taking machines apart and putting them back together again (sometimes they even worked). I spent my childhood cold and muddy, with the smell of petrol in my nostrils. When I was sixteen, my dad had bought me an old classic Mini to teach me car stuff before I was let loose into the world. That being said, I spent more time on the side of the road putting the exhaust back on, attempting to get the wipers going again, or reconnecting the battery leads than actually driving.

I'd never driven anything as big as the truck I'd now set my sights on, however, and had to quickly book a three-day intensive training course and test. The morning of the practical exam, the truck I'd trained in broke down and I had to swap to a different, longer vehicle. Somehow, I managed to pass with a clean sheet. Neither the examiner nor I could believe it. I had pulled off a similar last-minute trick for my motorcycle test as a broke university student. Being hell-bent on passing my test, I bought a cheap pair of handlebars off eBay and spent hours watching YouTube videos and walking round the garden of my student flat, pretending to check mirrors and indicate before changing 'lanes'.

After I totalled the Mini attempting a handbrake turn on ice (sorry, Dad!), I got a short-wheelbase, TD5 Land Rover

Defender. Aged eighteen, I packed it full of wetsuits and set off from Loughborough to Cornwall, where I tried to teach myself to surf. Each night I would head to a park-up, grab a sleeping bag, zip the suitcase underneath me shut and curl up into a ball in the back of the Landy. If you've ever been in the back of a short-wheelbase Defender, you'll know there isn't enough room to stretch out from the foetal position. But I was eighteen, and I didn't care one bit about using my suitcase as a mattress. I was living the dream!

After the Landy came a small Ford Transit Connect, and soon the weekend adventures became more regular, more scenic, more daring, and I definitely used up a couple of my nine lives.

I welded a metal frame to create a folding bed/bench seat, carpeted it with thick commercial carpets and added some superglued LED lighting to finish it off. My friends teased me, saying it looked like a failing bordello, but I loved it. Then there was the Volkswagen Transporter T5 I bought when I moved in with my then girlfriend, before the opportunity to buy a dirt-cheap ex-fleet-hire Mercedes Sprinter was too tempting to say no to.

This time around, I had the tools and builders' merchants accounts to make it a rough-and-ready, cheap, fast job. I was dead chuffed with the results. The sliding door opened to a bench seat with kitchenette, and I sacrificed a bathroom to make sure I had a big double bed sat over a compartment where I could keep a motorbike accessible from the rear doors. It looked rough on the outside, with only marker lights and an awning added to its pranged bodywork, but inside felt posher than a Scouser's hair salon with fake suede walls and roof, black glittery worktop and teak-finish cupboards.

It wasn't a show vehicle, but it wasn't meant to be. It was designed to get us from A to B very quickly on a Friday night, down tracks made for Land Rovers, past horribly scratchy bushes, and then to act as a rooftop bar, while we propped muddy push bikes and sandy surf boards up against it all weekend, before driving back home too fast halfway across the country late on a Sunday evening.

All the scratches, prangs and the faint outline of the previous hygiene company's logo on the back doors made it special. I've often found that too many people who do as we did overspend on the conversion and then, understandably, don't want to drive their expensive asset down narrow Cornish country roads, fighting past tractors and German campervans to find a parking spot. In my book, cheap, rough, and ready for action always wins.

The camper became a holiday villa for me and a bunch of mates who would pile surf boards, paddleboards, dogs and beer inside until we could barely shut the door, before driving off in search of remote beaches and wild mountains to explore. It was cheap and cheerful adventure and we all loved it.

It was on those wild weeks away, however, that I dreamt of a bigger vehicle – and a bigger trip. It was there where my desire for a truck was born.

Over the next few years, on and off, I would enquire, investigate specifications, make notes, and dream up how, once my little business made XYZ, we could sell up and go travelling. This was all to the absolute disapproval of my then fiancée, who at one point on a quiet Sunday night ended up crying and pleading with me to shut up about the whole thing. She was sick to death of hearing about it as I sat at the dinner table, notebook in hand, looking up the water capacity of a truck versus our van.

Now that I was newly single, nursing a broken heart, I realized this was the time to finally make my truck dream a reality.

I thought of Red and me roaring up steep mountain tracks, fording deep rivers, arriving at places no one else had been able to get vehicles to, then pulling out the barbecue, sticking up the fairy lights, having a hot shower outside and enjoying a cold beer in some of the most incredible scenery the world has to offer.

Nothing else would do. The dream had been born, the vehicle chosen, the lessons learnt – it was now time to get stuck in.

Once the business had been taken care of, I set about selling any and all personal items, from push bikes to surf boards, to old tools, even my old Mercedes Sprinter campervan, to be able to afford it.

My mum, seeing the dramatic U-turn in motivation, stepped down from suicide watch and decided to help kick-start this mad project. She didn't think I would actually pull it off, but reasoned that it would be a nice distraction, so very kindly offered to loan me the money to buy the truck.

I will forever be grateful for her support through my life. She has been my motivator, business adviser and confidante, and as things started to go wrong, she morphed into my relationship adviser, then counsellor.

Truck It!

So, on 15 May 2023, I drove a beat-up, old MAN truck to the farm and parked it proudly next to my caravan. My dad, whose natural northern scepticism had returned by this point after I sent him pictures, was very vocal about all the practical issues I needed to address. He has always been incredibly can-do, but often not when it comes to my latest hare-brained idea for some reason . . .

The campervan sale had given me enough money to start buying and fitting some parts, and I also painted it blue, cut windows in the back meant for horseboxes, and bought timber to build a bed frame. But I didn't have the money to finish the build, never mind actually set off driving anywhere.

Taking a leap of faith, I sold the caravan I had been living in for over a year and cleared a workbench of tools in a storage shipping container on the farm to use as my bed. Red slept each night on the floor surrounded by spare parts, tools and clothes packed in bags, while I climbed up to my sleeping bag, set up on a second-level wooden workbench, using a builder's lamp to see.

My dad came down from up north. His understandable scepticism fell away when he saw how committed to it I was. He got stuck in with sleeping on the floor of the truck, showering under the outside tap, and the two of us would often share a curry and a pint at the local Indian after a long day grafting underneath the oily adventure machine. Those times together I will never forget, and will be forever grateful for.

The final step towards freedom arrived when I eventually came out from behind closed doors, started my first Instagram page – having never done any social media before – and did a ten-second video announcing that I was selling all my worldly belongings, converting a truck to a home on wheels, to then take me and my best mate Red from England to Australia.*

Watching back that video, you can hear how lacklustre and hoarse my voice was. I was so tired, and still not back to being the full, bubbly version of myself.

For the next video, I used some old cardboard to draw a map of the world and the route I intended on taking, which at this stage was basically: go to France, head south and east *a lot*, to Australia.

These two videos went viral, but funnily enough, at this point, I had done *zero* prep. I had done no visa applications, no route-finding. Nothing, actually, other than buying a truck. I didn't know if what I was trying to do was even possible. But I didn't care. I was fully committed to getting on with it, and going as far as I could. I thought my chances of actually making it to Australia were slim, but I told myself over and over again that this was going to be about the journey, not the destination.

What an adventure it was going to be.

There was no turning back now.

---

* Personally I find talking about social media in a story like this a bit dull. Basically, just imagine that as well as everything else that's happening, I'm also trying to film stuff, keep cameras charged and reply to comments.

2

Bon Voyage

I was in the most beautiful place I had ever seen – sitting on the shore of an alpine lake so clear I had been able to see every detail of every stone fifty feet below me when I'd swum with Red that morning – and I couldn't stop crying.

We were in mainland Europe to test the truck for a couple of weeks while I waited for the sale of a site we'd developed that would give me the money to finish off the truck and pay for just about enough fuel and food to get me to Australia. The summer season had just finished and the plan was to drive up from the shores of Lake Annecy to the ski resorts in France and Italy.

For almost two weeks I had been driving around the Alps, Red on the passenger seat, head out of the window with his ears and big tongue flapping in the wind, stopping to swim in every clear river and lake I could, counting down the days until freedom, gorging on croissants and sipping fine Italian wine.

One evening, I sat outside enjoying the final moments of the light, playing with Red in a high mountain pasture, listening to the gentle clang of cow bells from cattle grazing in the next field and the odd marmot's chirp. The air was so clear and clean as I watched a red kite hover in the air overhead looking for prey. Under the painted blue sky, I dreamt of what was to come.

Aside from a vague start and end point, those two weeks were completely unplanned; I had no agenda. It was the first time I'd taken a break since my relationship had ended just over eighteen months previously, during which time every moment of every day had been taken over by some urgent deadline to do with the business as I battled in vain to save it. Even before that, as I'd been growing the business, I had put so much effort into being the boss, it had distorted who I was.

Now, it was as if we were going where the wind blew us, and I felt like I was just beginning to remember who I was. Before I'd left for this trip, I'd started to doubt if I was doing the right thing. I was at the stage of my life where I was supposed to be settling down, buying a house, starting a family. Instead, I was setting off on a glorified gap year. Shouldn't I give up on this, get a real job? That was certainly what some of the people who'd watched my videos thought. They were especially worried about Red.

You can't take a dog around the world . . . It's too dangerous for Red . . . he'll be attacked by the strays . . . You won't be able to pass through borders with him . . .

Truck It!

I knew I wanted my best friend with me but, if I was honest, they had a point.

Our experience of travelling together, Red and I, consisted of a lot of weekends camping in different campervans around the British Isles, from the outer Hebrides to the coast of Pembrokeshire, to surf weekends in Cornwall and fish-and-chip excursions down the east coast. Every now and then we would make a mad dash to France to spend a couple of weeks sunning it up for our summer holiday. He'd only just forgiven me for the time when, on one of those trips back from France, we'd stopped off at a rural vet for the mandatory worming tablet and health check, and without warning (or a glove) the vet put her finger up Red's arse. I'll never forget his facial expression. When she had finished, he squatted down, trying to make sure that, whatever happened, no one was doing *that* again.

Thankfully, we hadn't needed to visit any vets on our trip so far, and Red was loving the adventure.

In a beautiful little French village called Beaufort, I fell into an old, dimly lit shop full to the brim with teetering stacks of everything you could think of. I could barely speak any French, but it was of no concern to the eccentric, bubbly, bat-shit-crazy old French women, who found it hilarious that I was buying an old cow bell for Red as a joke. I managed to get across that I was about to drive to Australia with my dog, which she found just as hilarious, spending the next fifteen minutes talking *at* me while I giggled and laughed as I picked up the odd word, making hand gestures in response.

In Lacs Merlet, 2,500 metres up the Courchevel valley,

Bobby Bolton

Red and I were lounging on the banks of another alpine lake, the sun blazing down, a cool breeze whipping tiny waves onto the surface of the water, when a jolly old French man appeared over the mountain path, came down to the water's edge, where again he spoke *at* me playfully for a few minutes, before stripping off to reveal small white Y-fronts, half covered by his big overhanging belly. I watched, giggling, as he inched into the water, all the while making high-pitched shrieking noises at the cold, before he dived beneath the surface. Something about the big blue truck just seemed to grab people's attention.

In another alpine village, one old guy did a double take and walked back in my direction wearing a big smile with an outstretched hand to shake. 'What is this? . . . I have never seen something like this before . . . Where have you been? . . . Where are you going? . . . I don't believe you . . . that is incredible,' said Jean-Michel in a thick French/Belgian accent. He was in his early seventies and told me he had never grown up in the mountains and had only just recently started to hike by himself. He was now undertaking a solo hike, staying in remote huts over the next few days. We traded stories and as the conversation died off he insisted he be updated as the trip progressed. 'Do you have Instagram, Facebook, YouTube?' I asked, all of which he shook his head to. 'Okay,' I said, 'do you have an email address?' 'YES, I DO!' he shouted. So, I jotted it down, shook hands and watched him slowly shuffle off over the next rise.

For the first time in a long time, I could see the future stretching out in front of me.

Then the email arrived.

Truck It!

Dear Bob, I'm sorry but we have decided not to proceed with the sale.

Fourteen words – that's all it took. Without the money from the sale of the barn conversion, that was it. Dream over. I was due to start the drive back, but now it would be a funeral procession, not a victory march. I sat on the bank and stared into the water. Red came and sat next to me. I thought of returning back 'home', a shipping container on a derelict farm, where 'bed' was a tool bench and the bathroom was a Portaloo. Where I'd be washing in an outside tap and stealing electricity, which needed to be unplugged every morning before 7 a.m. when the neighbouring business turned up.

I had enough money left to my name for about six tanks of fuel, and no job to go back to. The only bright spot came in the Eurotunnel, when three German women walked past the open door of the truck, then a few seconds later came back and asked if they could have a look inside. They stood in the back of the truck, cooing at the fancy lights, full-sized shower and king-size bed. It turned out, they were on their way to a Christian festival in Sussex. After I told them about my plans for the trip, one of the women asked if she could bless me and the truck. She then spent almost five minutes blessing us while the whole group stood with their eyes shut. I'm not much of a believer, but even I had to admit it felt good to be on the receiving end of such a kind gesture from complete strangers. As she left the truck, she looked back over her shoulder and said, 'I can feel Jesus is looking over you, and he has a great big smile on his face.' I really hoped that was true.

I sheepishly made my way back to the farm, head in hands. From the sounds of things at the final site, it wasn't going to sell any time soon. An illegal caravan site had sprung up opposite and spooked every potential buyer. My dreams were dashed.

'Just come back home,' my mum said when I called to tell her I was home safe. 'I'm sure we'll be able to find you a job driving a digger or working for the local builder . . . You can stay in our spare room.'

The thought of that was absolutely crushing. I love my parents, and their support has been absolutely unwavering, but the idea of running back home to Mummy at this stage in my life was unbearable. Come hell or high water, I was going to pull this off.

I took selling the last of my belongings to a new level to squeeze every penny out of shirts, old PlayStations, old Land Rover parts, and anything eBay would allow me to post. I flogged axel stands, spare tyres, paddleboard paddles and had punters turning up at all hours of the day and night. Twenty quid here, fifty quid there – all of which went straight to the builders' merchants for a new grinding disc, a door hinge, or U-bend for the sink . . . I just had to keep going.

I reasoned that if I got rid of all of my personal items, my life would fit in the truck, thus severing every last tie to home, then surely something would have to give. Wouldn't it?

The videos I'd posted had started to get more and more views and comments, and I received loads of messages from people wishing me good luck, wishing they could do the same. People started copying in their friends – 'see, this is what we always said we'd do' – and then a message arrived that would suddenly start the countdown to lift-off:

Bobby, we would like to give you a free Channel Tunnel crossing to mark the start of your epic adventure.

It was from Le Shuttle (Eurotunnel) in Dover.

'That sounds awesome,' I replied. 'Does 30th September work?'

'All sorted, you're booked in,' came the response. 'See you soon.'

Amazing!

Only, at this point, I was far from properly prepared. Although I've found this is a tried and tested method to spur yourself on with achieving your goals. Sign yourself up for something, then you have to do it. It was a technique I'd used with running a marathon once. I signed up on the Wednesday and ran it on the Sunday with no training because I needed to prove to myself I could. This time around, however, I didn't even know if I was going to be able to cross the start line, never mind the finish.

The three-week countdown approached and another bit of good news arrived when sponsorship for the trip appeared from Kovered, a bag company that is owned and run by an old school friend. I was then separately contacted by a tracking company and one that sold e-bikes.

I couldn't believe it. I hadn't approached anyone, but as I'd posted more content from the build and the warm-up trip, it had caught the interest of some commercial enterprises.

The agreements were signed and my hopes of being able to pull this off were back with a vengeance. It would be by the skin of my teeth, but it was happening.

Bobby Bolton

I rang my dad two weeks out, with just over a thousand pounds, the truck, Red, and a few unsellable DVDs left to my name. 'Dad, I don't know what to do. I don't have the money to actually pull this off, but I'm stuck. I haven't told the sponsors I don't know how I'm funding the trip, but there's three signed up.'

'Listen. Just get on with it. You'll figure it out. If you have to stop and work somewhere for a while, then carry on, then you'll do that. Just get on with it. But first, make sure you come and say goodbye to everyone.'

With a week to go, I filled the long-range fuel tank I'd got second-hand off eBay and drove the five hours up north to see friends and family. My oldest and dearest friend, Ben, hosted a surprise gathering, and everyone signed an atlas with messages of support for what I was about to do. (They also, unbeknown to me, filled the truck with little gifts, pranks and sex toys, all of which I was to come across at very inconvenient moments over the coming months . . .)

I did a farewell tour of my hometown of Wigan and visited elderly relatives, including my Nan Irene, whose only comment bar 'hello' and 'goodbye' was, 'Ere, it's a bit big this truck, isn't it, Robert?' Her health was starting to go downhill and my dad said I needed to come and see her as she might not be alive by the time I got back. I hadn't realized just how hard it would be to actually leave.

But then the day arrived.

Luck, hard work, persistent sales, my ex buying me out of the flat and some inheritance money had, with a lot of compromises, just about finished the truck. I still had jobs to do as the Channel crossing deadline loomed, but there was no way I was delaying it. I knew if that date slipped, so would the dream of restarting my life.

Now, I'm the type of person who works well under pressure, but even having sold as many belongings as I had, packing up everything you will need to drive halfway around the planet into a truck in a single morning probably wasn't the smartest decision. I needed to leave at midday to catch the Eurotunnel at 3 p.m., but at 12.15 the bonfire I had started to burn all the wood offcuts and cardboard from the build was still blazing. I was desperately running out of time, so grabbed two handfuls of kit, threw open the doors of the container, and ran with my eyes shut and breath held, past the heat and smoke of the inferno, to the safety of the truck parked upwind.

Setting that alight at the last minute, where it was, was probably not the smartest decision I'd made in recent history, but certainly something I won't forget any time soon.

The fire was still burning as I neatened it up for the last time and prayed it wouldn't set fire to anything else while no one was around. I filled the water tanks, threw the jerry cans on the roof, lifted Red into the co-pilot position and, with a badly packed truck with items thrown in loose in the rear living area, set off to Dover as quick as I could.

My dad and his partner Karen had decided to make the journey from Wigan to Dover for the big send-off. We met at the nearest fuel station to the Eurotunnel, where he paid to fill the tanks with fuel.

'Have a ball. Have an absolute ball,' he said, hugging me as we both cried.

It was now time to spend some time with myself and work

out who I really was. After it so very nearly not happening, I still felt oddly hesitant. My confidence had been so knocked over the previous year or so, I kept thinking I'd have done something wrong, or forgotten something, and someone would come and tell me that of course I couldn't do this!

And yet even so, with just £600, a truck, a dog and a full tank of fuel to my name, I set off. This time for real.

3

Boy Meets Girl

I stood to admire the sun setting over the French Riviera, the high thin cloud orange against the darkening mountains. There wasn't another soul for miles.

Suddenly I heard a rustling in the bushes. My first thought was that Red had woken from his snooze in the truck and come to find me. I wondered if it was one of the local wild boar I'd been told about. But about two metres below me, out popped a beautiful white dog, followed by a gorgeous woman dressed in running kit, her hair tied up, headphones in. She stopped to admire the view, breathing heavily.

Holy crap, I thought. *She is stunning.*

I stood back out of view as the nerves and surprise of the moment took over. But then I gave myself a talking-to. *Come on, Bobby. Don't be shy. Say hello.*

'*Parlez-vous Anglais?*' was the best I could come up with in the moment.

'*Oui,*' she snapped back, somehow communicating that not only was it ridiculous that I thought that she might not be able to speak English, but that this was almost as ridiculous as the fact I couldn't speak French. She had tattoos on her arm and was looking at me fiercely.

I swallowed. 'I have a truck,' I said, gesturing vaguely back down the track. 'I'm driving it to Australia.'

She nodded.

'It's very beautiful here,' I said.

She nodded again and I got the feeling she wasn't up for a chat.

Sooner than perhaps I'd liked, I called out '*au revoir*' in my best French accent. She gave a quick half-wave without looking, then skipped back into the bushes, her dog following obediently behind.

That was un petit merde, *Bobby*, I said to myself.

I sat for twenty minutes with my legs dangling over the edge of the cliff, listening to the chorus of crickets getting louder as the last of the sun disappeared. Of course she hadn't wanted to talk to me. What was I thinking? But that didn't matter, I told myself. I needed to get used to relying only on myself. I could see the lights from the sailing boats twinkling in the distance as they rocked in the darkness. I was lost in my thoughts of what was coming.

I strolled back down to the truck, stuck the barbecue on, hung out the fairy lights and made a fuss of Red.

Later that evening, I opened my phone.

Truck It!

There was an Instagram message from a girl holding a small white puppy with big ears:

Cool truck.

It turned out the woman I'd met on the trail was called Marie. Rubia was the name of her dog.

After telling myself not to cock it up for a second time, I told her that my dog, Red, didn't know anyone and asked her whether Rubia would be up for showing him the local beaches.

'Okay,' she replied, 'sure.'

I couldn't quite believe my luck. She had seemed completely unimpressed, but now I was learning that she had been interested enough to take a quick picture of my Instagram handle, which I had painted on the truck.

The following day, I pulled over to the side of the road and up into the truck jumped this still very beautiful but now very smiley French woman, accompanied by her seemingly *huge* dog, and we all headed for L'Escalet beach a few miles outside of Saint-Tropez.

I owe serious wingman points to the truck, because for the duration of the ride, Marie smiled and wooed at driving in a vehicle that loomed over all other cars and drew loads of attention as we noisily made our way to the beach, mounting a few verges and curbs before releasing the hounds, who both ran straight into the water together.

'Well, at least the dogs get on,' I said, thinking that was a good sign. But at the back of my mind, I was wondering, *What exactly is the plan here?* I'd managed to talk my way into a beach date with a stunning French girl, but why? For a bit of company? The chance to socialize? I wasn't sure, but as we spent a few hours walking through the area, swimming with the dogs, she was incredibly easy to talk to.

I gave her the most upbeat-possible version of my year from hell, while she told me about growing up in Saint-Tropez, surrounded by the super wealthy, whom she had nothing in common with, and how she just wanted to go and spend time with her grandparents in the mountains. Her father was a semi-professional tennis player and she had won a tennis scholarship to go to college in America. Then she'd gone travelling around South America, learning Spanish, doing odd jobs and volunteering. She'd spent six deliriously happy months of her life working with horses in Argentina, but then Covid had forced her to return to France. She had felt pressured to settle down and work out a career, but she was clearly chafing at the bit and desperate to travel more. I didn't need to explain my trip to her at all. She got it immediately. We compared our lists of countries we'd always wanted to visit, laughing at how many times we said, 'Me too!' We joked that we should make a date to meet in South America when I was done with Australia.

'What are you up to tonight?' I asked over an ice cream on the way back to the truck.

'Actually not that much,' she said with a grin.

'Let me cook for you, then. I've got a couple of steaks in the fridge, a couple of bottles of local wine . . .'

She leaned back and let out a 'how ridiculous is this' kind of laugh before giggling her response: 'Sure.'

I couldn't believe it. I almost skipped back to the truck.

Truck It!

A few hours later, just before sunset, I met her and Rubia and apologized to Red as I threw Rubia in his direction with the instruction to 'Be friendly mate, it's only for a few minutes.'

I drove the four of us back up through the mountain tracks to the most perfect spot I had scouted out during 'shower time', before dressing in my best 'I'm wild and adventurous but still smartly dressed' outfit, which comprised of my least stained trousers and an actual shirt.

It was a quiet patch of flat sandy grass, only a few metres lower than the viewpoint, looking back over the same view that had brought us together twenty-four hours earlier. The fairy lights were strung up, barbecue warmed, a bottle of rosé retrieved from the fridge, and instructions given on how to cook the veg. She was surprised to be given orders, but giggled, picked up the knife and got stuck in.

The dogs played, wine flowed and laughter filled the warm, still night air while we cooked up a storm together, before cheers-ing and getting stuck in. As we ate, we poked fun at each other and told stories.

At one point she turned to me and said: 'I'm sorry I was in such a bad mood when we first met.'

I held out my hands to say no problem.

She went on: 'I was already in a bad mood because my boyfriend cancelled our weekend plans to go drinking with his friends and I was going to my special place, where I go to be alone, and there was this guy!'

'Well,' I said, 'I think your boyfriend is a very silly man.'

Having had my self-confidence completely shredded only a few months earlier, I couldn't quite believe I was here, in

France, having a beautiful evening with this funny, adventurous, outdoorsy girl.

One bottle of wine became three and a half, and we soon found ourselves lying on top of the truck's roof, stargazing into the night's sky.

Chris Stapleton's 'Tennessee Whiskey' played on the speakers and I hesitantly sang along as the conversation paused, mesmerized by the stars dancing above our heads, as we lay there under a blanket.

I turned to Marie, who seemed to have been wearing a permanent smile all evening, catching her eye before leaning in for a cheeky kiss.

As our lips touched, my heart skipped a beat. We both turned back to face the dark night sky, giddy, grinning like naughty teenagers. When it was time to get down from the roof, she half climbed, half fell as the dogs came to her rescue, licking her face.

'You can stay here tonight,' I said innocently half an hour later as the last bottle was finished. 'Absolutely no way,' she slurred. 'I'm going to walk home.'

'Marie, that's like over ten kilometres,' I protested, 'and it's half one in the morning – no way!'

I hopped into the truck and made up the 'spare bed'.

'Here, look, I'll sleep on the spare bed in the sleeping bag, and you can have the bed.'

'Nope,' she responded, shaking her head.

'Marie, you can't just sleep on the seat,' I said as I saw her eyes start to shut as she slouched in the camping chair I'd set up, one leg on the floor, one up and over the end.

I jumped back inside, got the cushions off the sofa/spare

bed, threw them on the floor outside the truck, and before I'd gone back in to retrieve cushions and a blanket, she was lying down, hugging her dog, who had lain down by her side.

I threw the blanket down, propped her head up on a cushion and, still wearing my boots, jeans and shirt, lay down next to her. I was just starting to drift off when, in a moment I won't forget, she rolled over and threw an arm over my chest before we both dozed off.

What a day. And what a woman.

All four of us woke only a few hours later at first light, as the sun slowly appeared on the horizon beyond the edge of the bay. Red had found a lovely little spot between my legs at the bottom of my bed, and had not budged an inch all night from a tight furry warm ball.

Rubia, however, had promoted herself to head of security and had, countless times in the night, set off at full sprint, barking as loud as she could into the nearest bushes. The last time, the sun was just coming up and I looked down at this beautiful woman with tousled blonde hair lying next to me.

That morning, after we'd had coffee, I dropped Marie and Rubia off at her car. We awkwardly hugged goodbye and I walked back to the truck with Red wagging his tail, head poking out of the window, saying goodbye to his new four-legged friend.

'Don't forget,' she said, just before we parted. 'Once you've finished in Australia, give me a call and I'll meet you over in Chile for another adventure.'

I laughed, staring back towards her crazy green eyes: 'You've got a deal.'

'See you in Chile.'

I dropped the handbrake, threw it into first gear, and set off towards the Ardèche river.

It was time for another adventure.

I spent the next couple of weeks cruising around France. Back when I had the campervan, a few times a year I'd set off to the French Alps at the last minute with a mate, the van full of tinned food and skis or paddleboards, depending on the season. We would take turns driving through the night, making sure we didn't sacrifice adventure time, before repeating the process, rolling straight off the Channel Tunnel at 4 a.m. Monday morning and going straight to work, our eyes blurred from no sleep and a busy weekend of adventures.

This time, however, I took my time cruising down scenic A-roads, rolling through the beautiful countryside of southern France, with the sun and sandy beaches of the south coast set as the destination for a much-needed few days' break to get my shit together. It took two days and lots of driving to reach the turquoise blue waters of the French Riviera, where I had been offered somewhere to stay for a few days by some extended family. Despite having only just set out on what I thought was to be an off-grid adventure, I reasoned that no one turns down a free holiday, so I gladly accepted, switched my phone off and spent a few days in holiday mode, walking along the beach, gawping at the boats in the bay of Saint-Tropez competing in Les Voiles.

My family filled up the diesel tanks, so once again, I was good to go for another few weeks. I'd spent the past few weeks looping back slightly north to explore areas I'd read about but hadn't yet visited on the first pass south.

Red and I spent a day paddleboarding thirty kilometres down the lazy-flowing Ardèche river, stopping to swim and snooze along the way. It was an incredible day of adventuring, and we returned to the truck by e-bike, having stashed Red's little trailer in a bush near the finish the day before. At sunrise the next morning, I finally got to see a cloud inversion over the sea from our mountain viewpoint, where the low lying cloud created a thick white fluffy blanket, hiding everything below us. If I noticed that I seemed to be circling the area of France where I knew Marie was, I didn't say anything. But when one day she messaged and asked if I knew anyone with a dog who liked paddleboarding, we agreed to meet up the following weekend at the Gorges du Verdon.

'See you there, can't wait,' she said. 'Make sure the rosé is in the fridge.'

The next day, Marie arrived in her mum's car with a big smile on her face, hugging me hello as the dogs started to play-fight.

We inflated two paddleboards, threw the dogs on and spent the day paddling across Lac de Sainte-Croix and up into the Gorges du Verdon, which have to be seen to be believed. The narrow gorge cliffs towered hundreds of metres straight out of the water. High overhead, huge buzzards circled rock climbers tackling some of the hardest and more notorious routes in Europe under the searing midday sun. Children climbed a few metres up the little rock and waterfall features, jumping, bombing and diving into the deep water as tourists in kayaks and pedalos ambled past.

The real gem, we worked out, comes at night, as all the hire shops closed and we meandered up the scenery alone, before returning to the glowing blue waters of the lake and back up to the truck parked along the shore.

We spent those two days joking, playing with the dogs, hiking up some aggressive but totally jaw-dropping mountains, driving up through winding mountain roads, stopping to buy local honey and sampling the regional food and wine.

Marie was up for anything and got stuck in, no matter how stupid the idea was. Whether it was scrambling up a rockface, dragging the dogs up behind us, running all the way back down along a mountain track, or actually having a go for the first time ever on a paddleboard and skinny-dipping in an ice-cold mountain river, she did it all with a smile and a spring in her step, before throwing a few insults and jokes in my direction. It was just so easy to talk to her and we saw the world in such a similar way. It felt more like I was reconnecting with an old friend than talking with someone I'd only just met. The past couple of days couldn't have gone better and this time she did stay the night inside the truck.

'Alright, well I guess this time I'll actually see you in Chile,' I joked as we embraced for a longer hug than the last.

'Have an incredible time,' she said as we parted. 'It's going to be absolutely epic.'

Okay, this is it, I said to myself. There would be no more tactical loops back towards her, nor was I prepared to cancel the trip for this girl, no matter how much I really liked her and how much we enjoyed each other's company. I had just left an eleven-year relationship. I obviously wasn't going to fall for the first pretty woman who said hello to me. This trip was about me, going solo, working out who I was. And now it could properly begin.

'*Au revoir*,' I shouted as she drove off down the road, waving back at me.

Red sat watching me carefully as I craned my head to see her in the mirror.

'Mind your own business,' I said in response.

4

The Italian Job

'Six days in?! Bobby, what the hell?!'

My mate Max had nearly spat his beer out when I told him about meeting Marie. He wasn't even smiling.

'Dude, that is too soon. You've literally just set off.'

Max and I had known each other for years after meeting at university and immediately bonding over our shared love of drinking beer and doing adventurous stuff like climbing up and abseiling down very high things. He'd fancied a slice of the action, so flew out to the Dolomites to meet me for a mini adventure.

'Yeah, but what a story,' I said. 'Heartbroken Englishman and dog set off for the far side of the world to restart his life. Meets beautiful outdoorsy French girl, also with dog, BY SHEER CHANCE up the top of a mountain. They fall in love, drive off into the sunset and live happily ever af—'

'Mate, this isn't a movie,' Max interjected. 'Can you actually imagine anyone in their right mind who would move in together after six days and one date?! Because that's effectively what you'd be doing.'

He had a point.

And he wasn't finished: 'So you'll be adding all this stress to a new relationship by trying to travel round the world with two dogs, which by the way you don't know is even possible in all the countries you need to get through.'

I held my hands up. It was a fair cop. He was right. He was always right, apart from that one night at university, when he woke me up at 3 a.m., standing outside my bedroom window, wearing only torn boxers and a pair of trainers, holding a six-foot staff made of taped-together beer cans, by shouting (loud enough to wake the whole street), 'SPARTAAAAAAAAAAA!', before projectile vomiting all over my van. Then, he had been wrong.

'It's not going anywhere anyway,' I said, swilling my beer around in my glass. 'She's in the middle of buying a house, so she's going to move in with her boyfriend. And she's just started a diploma thingamajig.'

'Sounds like that's that then, mate,' said Max.

'Silly bastard doesn't even like her dog,' I added.

Max patted me on the shoulder. 'Another round. Tonight, we drown your sorrows. Tomorrow, we'll climb Piz Boè.'

I nodded in agreement, necked my pint and walked to the bar.

I nearly hadn't made it to Max at all. I had been weirdly

nervous as I was about to cross the border from France into Italy in the late October sunshine. I felt like I knew France a bit. I'd gone there as a kid, driven my campervan there over the past few years. And in terms of food, I could get by with my tourist French. But Italy would be the first time I was taking the truck into a country I knew almost nothing about. I'd been once, with my mum skiing, but it would be the first place I'd visited, other than France, on my own.

Things hadn't started brilliantly when I'd snapped the sub chassis coming over some rough off-road ground in a gorge. However, without the budget to pay for a professional repair, I bought fifty euros worth of metal flat plate from a metalworker's yard, parked at a quiet spot by a river next to the border and set about cutting, drilling and bolting a splice plate. It was hard graft, but it worked, and I was thankful for my dad's advice to take some essential tools just in case. So, I crossed the border nervous but on a high.

I set my sights on a spot in the mountains near Turin, which turned into an epic three-day off-road adventure, having accidentally stumbled across an almost one-hundred-mile, high mountain track where apparently people from all over Europe flock to in the summer. It was the most incredible, high and winding route through the mountains, at the same height as the clouds, with views all down the valleys.

I stopped the truck and looked down at the border between France and Italy, and in the other direction was Switzerland. Crossing into Italy, I ended up at another mountain, this time the Matterhorn, where I spent a whole day exploring closed ski runs with Red in tow, through fresh snow. We

Truck It!

hiked up to just over 3,000 metres and skied right back down to the door of the truck.

Mountains turned to lakes as I left the Alps behind, pointing east towards where I would be meeting Max. Before that, I decided to go via the famous lakes of Italy.

An odd thing happened, though, the further east I found myself driving. What had been wide open roads began to shrink. The cars too. Trucks, SUVs and four-wheel drives all turned to, almost completely without exception, Fiat Pandas. I felt as if I was Alice and had drunk the wrong potion. Who knows whether the cars are made small because of the small roads, or the other way around. All I know was that it was starting to feel a bit tight for my blue truck. It was a relief to park up on a dead-end section of road on the shores of Lake Orta as the light faded. A couple of hours later, I was sat in darkness with the side door open, enjoying a beer, when a car turned up to what they must have thought was a quiet, romantic spot. They parked five metres in front of the truck and Red pricked his ears up at the unmistakeable sounds of two people 'enjoying' each other's company. I left it for a bit, but when it became clear they weren't finishing any time soon, I crept into the cab, turned the ignition on and activated the four, what can only be described as NAVY search-and-rescue spotlights, each one brighter than the sun.

Limbs went flying, clothes were grabbed and, as I sat crying with laughter, tyres screeched and the two lovers hurtled off down the road. It took me five minutes before I could move for laughing. What's Italian for *in flagrante*?

I spent the next couple of days winding around the great lakes of Italy, stopping at Maggiore, Lugano and Como. Each lake has a slightly different character, with multicoloured villas and palaces dotting the hills crowded with cypress, laurel and palm trees, all the way down to the water's edge. There was no way I could get through the traffic in the truck, so I'd park up on the outskirts and take the bike out for coffee and a pastry. At Lake Como, I took Red out on the paddleboard past the arches and vaults, the water a rich green underneath us. Even though it was late October and overcast, it was still heaving with tourists, taking boats across the lake, wandering through leafy promenades, or cycling up and down the shores. I'd spent the day with Red, lazily swimming, walking and sipping overpriced Italian coffee, dreaming of how I'd be as a rich seventy-year-old retiree.

George Clooney's home here is said to be worth $100 million. But would I swap it for my big blue palace? (Yes, yes I would.)

On one of my swims, I'd spotted an overnight wild camp spot, high above the west shore.

Up there, I thought, *out of the hustle and bustle. Hopefully the roads have been widened for tractors and forestry work.*

I shuffled, cursed and honked my way through the last of the narrow lakeside villages where the truck's tyres literally scraped the front step of someone's house, while the other side clipped a parked-up Fiat Panda. I was quickly learning that the Italian style of parking was to abandon your car anywhere there was space. Some locals cursed and made stereotypical hand gestures, signifying, I think, 'What a beautiful truck, welcome to our country', but I could be wrong.

Half an hour later, halfway up the hill and with Lake Como stretching out below me, I paused to take it all in. It was by

Truck It!

any measure an extraordinary view. But there was a little voice in my head saying, 'Yeah it's goooood, but we're only halfway up. I wonder if we can get all the way up to the top . . .'

Now, this tendency to ask 'what if' is a curse I've had ever since I first started exploring in a campervan and which I'm yet to find a cure for. It's led to some amazing adventures over the years, but it's also landed me in some sticky spots. At this moment, it was saying, 'Yes, sure, this is a pretty cool view, the perfect spot to park, but look, there's a muddy, stony track leading up that steep hill, maybe we can go to the very top and get an even better view. Keep going, Bobby.' So off we went.

The track at the start was pretty good, with about a quarter of a metre spare either side of the truck, flanked by a gentle bank. Easy. But about half a kilometre later, the track doubled back on itself into the wood. It became clear there was no way I could make that turn. Would I have to drive back down? I paused momentarily to assess my options.

Directly ahead of me was another track, unmaintained, with fewer stones, slightly narrower, flanked by steep banks either side. What if I went that way?

I set off, dropping the truck into a low ratio as I pulled up my phone to see if this track would bring me back up to the track I had just—

My heart dropped.

I grabbed the steering wheel, braced and gritted my teeth, and jumped as hard as I could on the footbrake.

After what felt like an hour as time stood still, the truck juddered to a stop.

I opened the door and saw the rear right wheel hanging

off the bank, which was so steep it fell away like a cliff. Mud and debris had fallen down the steep drop and the truck was leaning seriously to the side.

Shiiiiiiiit. How did that happen?

I climbed out of the cab, swinging around the bumper to avoid falling down the bank, given this second track had narrowed down so severely it was now only a little over the width of the truck. Of all the stupid homages to *The Italian Job* . . .

The ground was saturated as I walked around to find the culprit – a big rock sticking out of the ground which had made the truck jump and the track on the lower side collapse. Head in hands, I went round the back to see that the truck was now completely resting on its belly, with one wheel floating in the air. I'd been incredibly lucky that the whole thing hadn't just slid backwards down the hill. I grabbed onto saplings to climb down below the bank and take in the full picture. A tree root had caught one of the lockers just in front of the rear wheel, which had fortunately taken the weight and was holding it in place.

At this stage, I felt bullish. I had four-wheel drive, brand-new, top-of-the-range tyres from Continental Tyres. *Bring it on*, I thought. So I climbed back up the hill and jumped into the cab.

At that moment, a hunter appeared from down the muddy forest track ahead of me, gun over his shoulder, dogs in tow. I watched him take in the truck. Then he came to the door and in loud, animated Italian told me that I probably shouldn't be reversing down a hill into Lake Como. My attempts to explain I didn't speak Italian proved pointless, so all I was

Truck It!

left with was a sheepish shrug to try to communicate that I'd cocked up. Though I couldn't understand the words he was using, I was pretty sure from the tone that he wasn't saying, 'You are a clever man and I like you'.

But I had a plan. I gestured for him to stand back as he took out his phone to take some pictures. I locked all the differentials, built the revs right up to the red line, and dropped the clutch.

The truck sent out a big plume of black smoke, violently shook, threw some mud around . . . but we didn't budge. Over the next five minutes, while I was inspecting the even bigger shit I'd just made for myself by digging three more holes under the wheels still on the track, Mr Angry took photos, rang various mates and even FaceTimed as he walked around the truck giving a running commentary. He then walked away shaking his head, laughing the whole way until he disappeared from view. At no point had he offered any form of help.

At that point, I rang my dad – who told me to send some photos. When he hadn't called me back after five minutes, I started to despair. I imagined having to call him to come and help me. Then it started to rain.

After ten minutes of listening to the sound of the rain in the trees, I decided I had to wipe the smile off that Italian hunter's face.

So, I devised a plan.

Stage one: try to cut down two chunky saplings with a blunt bow saw. Stage two: get pissed off at how long it's taking. Stage three: climb up half cut-down tree and, grabbing hold of a branch, jump off with full weight pulling down, attempting to save time. Stage four: tumble down a steep slope backwards before landing upside down against a tree and calling out 'I'm alive!' for the camera set-up, still filming where I had been. After checking to make sure I hadn't broken anything, I climbed back up the steep slope. The jack was in play. I tried jacking from different points around the back of the truck, but each time I set the jack up, it sank into the sodden ground before the truck even moved an inch. It was soul-destroying.

By this time it was pitch black and the four external floodlights were casting cones of white in the torrential rain. As the rain made the ground softer, the upturned ratchet bar I was using to pump the jack using maximum effort for minimum reward started to cut my hand.

I sat in the rain, defeated. But then, suddenly, I remembered Geoff, my dad's oldest and dearest friend, had insisted I take some old bits of wood that he'd cut up for me. Not wanting to be rude, and thinking that, if for no other reason, they would be good for firewood, I'd taken them with me. Now, those sixteen blocks could be the key to my freedom.

Over the next couple of hours, as midnight fast approached and all my clothes became soaking wet, I lay under the truck, cranking the jack and throwing a block of wood in each hole the jack made until, after about six blocks, the truck finally started to lift.

The elation I felt the first time the truck moved one centimetre upwards was massive, and I couldn't contain a primeval scream into the empty darkness of this wet, cold and miserable mountain forest.

Stopping only for a honey baguette for dinner and blasting

Truck It!

out AC/DC to keep my morale up, midnight came and went. The truck lifted enough so the floating wheel had enough space against the bank to place one block, then two, then four, until the bank that had collapsed was now built back up in a muddy mess. It was completely piss-wet-through and structurally unsound, but just about holding the wheel up.

Now what? The wheel was still over the edge of this bank, but the axle was not far off being level, marking significant but hard-earned progress. Even so, I couldn't reverse and I couldn't go forwards. At this point, my decision not to bring a proper hydraulic winch seemed to be a poor one. All I had was a Tirfor hand-cranked version. My dad had reasoned: 'If you ever get stuck enough to use this, you'll probably be screwed anyway and need the army to pull you out. Go for the £120 hand crank.'

I scrambled onto the roof and grabbed it, then strapped an extra rope for safety to the front of the truck to the best tree I could find. It was only rated up to three tonnes, so I wouldn't be able to winch the full weight of the truck on its own, but it would hopefully stop it sliding down the hill.

After some false starts, I lifted the rear axle up centrally and offered a prayer to the jack: 'I'm so sorry to put you through this, mate. Don't tell my dad, and please don't bend, please, otherwise we are all properly in trouble.'

I scrambled out from underneath the truck on my belly, tried to rid my hands of the worst of the mud, grabbed the winch handle and started pumping and pulling over the back of the truck towards the uphill bank. It worked! The truck had lifted and then moved. The floating wheel was now a whole lot closer to the track. Another wolf howl of triumph.

Over the next few hours, I jacked, propped and pulled as much as I could. Red refused to get out of the truck, but from time to time would come and watch. Eventually, all four wheels were back on the track. But there was no way I could drive across the collapsed track. So, using the trees I had felled earlier, a stack of blocks and two recovery boards, I made something the army logistics core would have been proud of. Would it take the weight of the truck, built on soaking mud? I had no idea, but would soon find out.

I unfastened the front safety line, dragged all the tools out of the way, kicked the mud off my boots, hopped in the truck and started her up.

'Please work, please work . . .'

My voice was hoarse from effort, dehydration and tiredness. My arms and hands were beginning to cramp with exhaustion from jacking and throwing heavy bits of wood around for what was approaching eight hours in wet mud.

Here we go!

I engaged four-wheel drive, locked the differentials and forced it into reverse.

I eased backwards, praying out loud we'd make it. The rear wheels made it across as I held my breath – then the front wheels. There was a loud crack as one of the trees beneath me gave way, but I punched the accelerator and as the front of the truck began to drop, the momentum was enough that we were dragged backwards as the bridge gave way. My final wolf call of the night ended in a cough, as the cold and exhaustion caught up with me and the adrenaline wore off. Red stirred momentarily in his bed next to me and half opened one eye to look in my direction before snoozing off.

I pulled out my phone, which was by this point absolutely caked in mud, wiped the screen with a corner of my wet T-shirt, and recorded a video in front of the spotlights, the rain coming down all around me. I was shaking from exertion.

I reversed the truck back to the junction where the curse had kicked in, left all the blocks, boards, snapped trees, tools, jack and wet muddy boots strewn over the bank and sank onto my bed, immediately falling asleep. I woke a few hours later so I could try to repair as much of the damage from last night as possible. I cleared away all the kit and, just as I was done, who should arrive but the Italian hunter. He wasn't in his hunting gear, but he was wearing a very surprised face. As I stood on the roof of the truck, I watched him walk around the truck. Then he just started clapping. I climbed down and he shook my hand with a big bear-like paw, before walking back off into the woods, still shaking his head.

It was the best reaction I could have asked for. I puffed my chest out, closed the last of the lockers and set off back down into the circus of Pandas, in need of a much-deserved coffee.

A week later, and it had become a story to tell for laughs, as Max and I skied and hiked our way through the thick snow of the Dolomites. The type of rock the mountains are formed of means that you get these incredible vertical outcroppings and steep valleys. It's almost like you're surrounded by skyscrapers. It felt amazing to spend time with such an old mate and think about nothing but the next adventure. I didn't tell him that I'd polled my followers that first night we'd got drunk and asked them if Marie should join the trip. 'Go for it' had won over 'don't be a plonker' by a slim margin: 57 to 43 per cent. Thousands voted and, to my amusement, emotions were high as followers sent strongly worded messages in favour either way.

A few days later, I dropped Max, my relationship adviser, off at the airport and headed to Lake Garda to thaw out. Sat with my feet dangling over the edge of a jetty on the eastern shores, throwing sticks in the water for Red, my phone dinged. It was Marie.

OK Bobby.

I can't stop thinking of you or the trip or Red!! It cannot stop after one weekend (at least I don't want it to).

Life gives you opportunities for you to take. I am taking mine . . . we have one life. I would love to invite myself and truck it with you!!

It might be too straight to the point, no rush and if you rather make it to OZ alone with Red; we will wait for Chile.

I read the message several times, wanting to make sure there was nothing that might have been lost in translation. Fifty-five minutes later exactly, having gone for a slow walk to calm the adrenaline, nerves, and to quickly confer with the Oracle (my mum), I responded:

Fuck it, let's do it.

I'm trusting in Fate.

5

What's French for 'Detour'?

'Marie, I said three bags!!' I teased, laughing as she knelt on the bed surrounded by a mountain of clothes and enough jars, lotions and potions to start a pharmacy.

'It is three bags,' she replied. 'Just three very well-packed, very big bags.'

It had been three weeks since Marie had seen my message and immediately called me. She told me she would tell her (now ex-) boyfriend to collect his stuff and clear off, ring her solicitor and cancel the house purchase. She then took herself off the scholarship programme she had just started to become a sports coach, much to the displeasure of the staff, who threatened her with all sorts, including the promise she would never be able to work in sport again.

'Well, we better not muck this up then,' I laughed.

'Seriously, though,' she said, 'I'm going to bring my tent. I don't want you to feel obliged to take me anywhere if it doesn't work between us. This is great but I really don't want to ruin your trip if it doesn't go well.'

I thought again how wild it was that I'd randomly bumped into someone so aligned with the way I saw things. She was prepared to drop everything at a moment's notice, rolling the dice on everything, all while calmly planning for the eventuality of it all going wrong. 'And if it doesn't work but you don't want to tell me, just leave my tent and dog lead outside the truck and I'll get the message,' she said. I looked at her and saw that she was serious. I told her exactly the same thing. Let's both be completely honest with each other. And if we ever need to have that conversation, we will.

We'd agreed to meet in Genoa, right on the border of France and Italy, which meant a loop back for me. The night before we were due to meet, I'd arrived in a newly cleaned truck with fresh sheets, neatly packed clothes cupboards, and a brushed-out driver's cab complemented by the best fake pineapple air freshener to make the front smell like a public toilet. I decided to spend the night in the hills behind the city away from the hustle and bustle of the busy port city.

The sign read NO TRUCKS, with a big picture of a truck and a massive red cross through it. Now you might have thought that was easy to interpret, but I had learnt that, in Italy, locals often put their own signs up to dissuade noisy brutes from passing through their quiet but perfectly safe and legal streets. I decided this was definitely one of those ones. So, I inched the truck along the cobbles of the quaint mountain hamlet I had decided to stay in. I turned the ninety-degree bend into the centre, where a historic-looking stone archway stared back at me. *Shit. That's too small.* 'Wait, is it?' said the curse, nudging forward towards it.

Faces started to appear as shutter doors opened in the stone terraced houses at the sound of a large engine revving. My trusty blue companion had many strengths. When it was hauling us up steep mountain tracks or making short work of crossing a river, it was in its element. But here, nudging our way through narrow streets, lined by houses, I felt like an elephant trying to do ballet. Aware of the many pairs of eyes watching me, I decided that I couldn't admit defeat. Again, that little voice said, 'Sure, it'll be alright . . .'

I reasoned that I'd just take it really slowly and if I heard the smallest of contacts with the arch, I'd stop immediately. I knew that the spot I'd found where I could park up was just over the next hill. To go around the hamlet would add more than an hour. My first mistake was not stopping when the stone pillars pushed both wingmirrors closed. Not only did that mean I couldn't gauge if we were going to fit, I also didn't know if we were in the middle of the arch. Still, in for a penny . . .

I edged forward at a snail's pace, holding my breath to be as quiet as I could, to hear if the truck made contac—

And then there was a sound like the sky had fallen in.

The truck rocked and the roof bent in menacingly. Plumes of dust rose. I tried to open the doors, but they were pinned shut. I reasoned something must have collapsed on us, but what? I slowly backed out, at which point I saw that half the historic arch was missing, or, rather, was now in pieces on the truck.

I'm not proud of it, but my first instinct was to quietly drive away. My Italian wasn't good enough to say, 'I thought your sign saying "No Trucks" was fake, but now I see it is real and I am truly sorry I have demolished your beloved local monument'. However, the growing crowd of pissed-off-looking locals made that highly unlikely. There was about fifty of them and they were just beginning to get that 'where did I put that pitchfork?' look to them. I reversed slowly around to a gravel car park where I was marshalled to stay by angry locals. One of them spoke enough English to tell me to say there until the 'mayor' arrived. I wasn't sure whether or not to feel relieved that it wasn't the police. While I waited, I decided to take a look at the damage I'd done. There were about a dozen ancient hand-carved blocks resting on the roof of the truck. I moved them gently, wincing as I saw that they'd bent the frame of the solar panel, but offering silent thanks that they didn't seem to have damaged the panel itself.

I thought how, only two days before, I had been in the Dolomites with Max and Red. We had parked up and hiked up into the mountains. The landscape had been like something from another planet, the dark rock jutting up out of the gravel and ice, like the sides of a cathedral.

Then the snow and mist had properly come in, all sound muffled by snow, Red shaking the fat flakes from his fur in a mixture of irritation and delight.

The original plan had been to pack climbing kit, shorts, shades and caps, which, given it was approaching the end of October, was slightly optimistic in hindsight. The once dry, beautifully green rolling hills with rock spires reaching high into the sky had turned into white blankets. Shorts were left neatly folded in Max's suitcase, and I dug out what spare winter kit I had.

In typical Bobby and Max fashion, the damp November blizzard weather didn't hamper our enthusiasm for climbing these incredible rock features, nor Red. It was a resounding success as we just about managed to cling to mountain sides before we both almost lost a couple of fingers to frostbite on our last day.

The highlight had to be rescuing a pair of rather emotional middle-aged men with a small white fluffy dog in tow from a snow blizzard as their car was stuck and they dared not even set foot outside. We also explored abandoned caves that the Italians had used during the Second World War to conduct mountain warfare. They had been cut by hand and took impossible routes through the mountains, up sheer rock faces, popping out hundreds of metres overhead. They were pitch black and smelt dank and at points narrowed until you had to crawl on your belly over the wet stone. It was incredible to think how only just over seventy years ago, they would have been full of soldiers, fighting and dying.

We bounced around, with no real plan or agenda, just seeing where the wind blew us. It was exactly what I wanted the trip to be about. Unfortunately, I had then bounced straight into this arch.

Through sign language and tone of voice, I managed to convey that I wasn't running away but just wanted to go and look at the site of the accident. Not only had the stonework and render come down from the top half of the arch, but the same could be said of the building next to the arch, leaving just the red brick of the structure underneath. One local was watching me particularly fiercely.

'Should have had the height up there, I reckon,' I said, gesturing weakly. But it was no good. We all knew who was at fault. It was the lemon with an enormous truck who'd tried to drive it through a local landmark. At that point, a guy in his early fifties arrived in a Fiat Panda (of course), jumped out and looked at the arch. I had been expecting all sorts of drama, but he calmly assessed the damage and then spoke quickly to some of the locals, who ran off. Then he came and shook my hand. He explained that they would need me to stay while they took photos of my documents, spoke to the town's lawyers and made the area safe. After they calmly helped to lift the enormous stone that had lodged itself behind my cab, the mayor shook my hand again and walked off. I could see why he was the mayor. I wanted to vote for him and I didn't even live here. I wondered for a moment what would have happened back home if an Italian bloke in an enormous truck had reversed through the Roman bathhouse in Wigan. Chaos. Utter Chaos.

I'd told the mayor I was a builder and would be in the area for a few days if they needed me to stay and help repair the arch. Though, I didn't tell him my rendering skills were pretty much non-existent. After waiting a respectful few minutes, as the locals began dutifully piling stone by the side of the road, I called out 'cheers then', and drove away to find the spot on the main mountain road I'd been looking for. The difference between up in the mountains, where the blue truck had been our passport to another world, and civilization, where it had all come crashing down, couldn't have been starker. I spent that night expecting to get a knock on the door and be presented with an enormous bill.*

All this meant I was still a bit amped the next morning when I drove down into Genoa to meet Marie. There was absolutely nowhere I was going to be able to park in the city, so after I'd had to leave the third full car park, I ditched the truck in the middle of a T-junction, while Marie's mum abandoned her car as close as possible to minimize the ferrying back and forth. Neither my French nor her English were up to the task, so I tried to signal that I was exactly the sort of person who she could trust to look after her daughter, and she tried to impress, mainly through gestures, that I'd better not be a serial killer, as Italian motorists honked their horns ever more enthusiastically around us. It took about four minutes and then suddenly Marie was calling out *'Bisou'* as they kissed and she ran off. There was just time for a parking attendant to have arrived on a moped, and start writing out a ticket. 'It's okay, we're leaving!' I called as we tried to load the dogs into the truck – neither of whom were particularly impressed that there was currently only one single plywood box bed.

Keen to escape the crowds, I drove up into the mountains as I explained to Marie why I had to avoid one particular

---

* I never did find out about the fate of that arch. I got a call a few months later from a disappointed-sounding guy from my insurance company, but nothing ever came of it, and I even got my proof of no-claims bonus when the policy finally ended.

route. She listened with mounting horror and then laughter as I told her the story of the previous night. I was keen to find somewhere tranquil and calm where we could all catch our breath and work out what would happen next. But I noticed that the streets were again beginning to get tighter and tighter the higher we went, with rows of parked/abandoned Fiat Pandas on either side of the road. Then, just as we made it through the final hamlet, the traffic coming towards us started beeping and the drivers gesturing.

'What's the matter?' said Marie.

'Don't worry, they're just Italian,' I said.

But soon, even I started to wonder what had happened, so I stopped and got out of the truck. At which point, I saw the builder's extension lead caught on the truck that we'd been dragging behind us, presumably since that builder we'd driven past about ten minutes ago. An angry Italian man leaned out of his Fiat Panda and shouted, probably telling me how fantastic the truck looked in blue, I think. I called out my thanks and untangled the extension lead. I weighed up jogging back down the hill with it before deciding it would be better for everyone if I left it somewhere obvious.

'All okay?' asked Marie.

'Yeah, lot of fuss over nothing,' I said. I didn't think Marie's faith in my driving could survive another snafu, however minor.

An hour later, we were parked up high in the mountains over Genoa and, over a beer, we traded stories about how everyone we knew thought we were crazy. We watched the Mediterranean Sea, flickering orange as the sun sank into it. I thought again how easy it was. How there were no nerves, or awkwardness. It was as if no time had passed between us. We just jumped straight back into the same dynamic as a few weeks before.

'So, where do you fancy going next?' I asked.

'Wherever. Just not back to Plan-de-la-Tour. I think my ex or solicitor might kill me if they see me,' she laughed.

'Yeah, and I need to get away from Genoa.' She clinked her bottle of beer against mine at that. 'So I reckon southern Italy, Austria or Slovenia.'

She shrugged and yawned. 'All sounds good.'

I thought again how life revolves around such small moments. Like the twenty seconds it took me to call down to Marie on that mountain top. She could so easily have run back into the scrubland before I'd said anything and left me alone with the sunset, wondering what might have been. It took twenty seconds to change my life, and I seized the moment.

We sat and watched the sun disappear as the dogs grumbled and then finally settled down next to each other.

6

Slovenia, I Hardly Knew Her?

'Hellooo! Can you help us?'

A loud French voice came echoing from high above. I turned to Marie. She had an ice axe in one hand, rope attached to Rubia in the other, wearing a climbing harness, purple sunglasses, a helmet, and was standing shin-deep in snow. We both looked at each other and scowled as the dogs pointed their ears back up the steep tracks we had all just roped down. It had been hard enough getting down, never mind going back up.

We were over 2,800 metres above sea level in the Julian Alps in Slovenia and had been climbing since sunrise, up into low cloud which had set on fire as the sun crept over the horizon just after 6 a.m. Neither of us had slept well the night before. Rubia had decided to wake up every time she heard a sound in the mountain hut we were staying in. But in the early morning light, the hut, which resembled a big garden shed perched on the edge of a cliff, had uninterrupted views for hundreds of metres down over the snow-covered valley, which was punctuated with towers of dark grey limestone. Max had told me that if we got a chance to go to Triglav National Park, we had to visit it. Even if it was officially too late in the year to climb, and all of the tracks and mountain refuge huts were closed.

And so Marie and I had both decided on that, rather than southern Italy. We'd started out east, aiming to cross the top of the boot of Italy and into Slovenia, which nestles in between Austria to its north and Croatia to its south. This was in spite of the fact that Marie had last skied fifteen years ago as a child on a family trip, had never held a climbing rope or put on a harness, and admitted to not really liking even going up ladders. I assured her, however, that I'd give her a crash course in mountaineering for beginners.

First, we stopped off a hundred kilometres east of Genoa at what is known as the Cinque Terre, which are five beautiful fishing villages of Riomaggiore, Manarola, Corniglia, Vernazza and Monterosso, perched on the hillside looking down over the Ligurian Sea.

The only problem was that when we arrived, we were told the coastal path was closed.

'Ah, I'm sure it'll be fine,' I said.

Cue a montage of us waist-deep in the rough breakwater, 'caving' underneath the foundations of an enormous wall, then over huge blocks of concrete as the waves smashed around us. Somewhere high above us were the jumble of multicoloured houses the villages are famous for. But instead of appreciating all that scenery, we were too busy climbing then abseiling, with the dogs on my shoulders, only to finally pop out cut, bruised and soaking wet, much to the bemusement of the American tourists getting stuck into their gelato. Marie didn't once complain. Instead, she just got stuck in, earning the highest available compliment from my mum – that Marie is a 'proper chap' – when I told her that evening. After that, I thought we all deserved a bit of luxury, so we decided to stop off for a day in Venice.

We parked up at a campsite in the mainland, got our glad rags on (easier said than done in a truck), then the four of us explored one of the most romantic cities in the world. Sixty years previously, my grandparents had visited Venice for their honeymoon. In the Basilica di San Marco (which sounds far more glamorous than St Mark's church), I took a Polaroid of the moment I asked Marie to be my girlfriend and she said yes. We kissed and giggled. This romantic moment was only slightly spoiled by the fact I hadn't checked to see if there was any film in the camera. Then we went for a celebratory drink. As we strolled back through the city, we arrived at the jetty on the Grand Canal we had been dropped off at, only to find that we had missed the last boat back to our campsite. No matter how many obscenely expensive taxis we tried to negotiate with, none would take 'two small well-behaved dogs'. So, we sprinted to the train station and hopped on a carriage as the doors were shutting. Upon arriving at an unknown location, we fired up Google Maps and, taking a deep chest full of air, started to jog in the direction of the truck, wearing the most inappropriate running clothes.

Truck It!

Marie panted, laughed and complained tongue in cheek all the way home. Rubia ran ahead with a spring in her step, barking at anything that moved as we made our way through dark industrial estates, while Red lagged behind, cursing with every laboured step. What better way could there be to celebrate Marie and I formally becoming a couple than doing no research, getting caught out, blagging it and finishing the day laughing our arses off?

After all that excitement, it was then a 150-kilometre drive east into Slovenia and north up to our first stop at Lake Bled, a glacial lake the shape of a giant teardrop. There, surrounded by snow-capped mountains, and surrounded by dark forests of spruce, fir, oak and pine, with the faint chiming of bells from the church that sits on an island in its centre, I found a suitable boulder and took Marie through more mountain techniques we'd need if we were going to make it up Triglav, the highest mountain in Slovenia. Yet again, I was struck by how nothing seemed to faze Marie. Within an hour, she was hanging off the boulder grinning, and another half an hour later, you'd think she'd spent her entire life climbing. Then, a couple of days later after a relaxed drive, we arrived at the National Park. As I switched off the engine, I turned to her.

'Ready to climb your first mountain?'

'Be gentle with me,' she said.

We hiked, climbed and scrambled through alpine forest, along cliff edges, passing through cloud inversions at sunrise, wading through waist-deep snow-covered tracks. To be doing all this with a woman I had spent barely a few days with was surreal. But it felt as if we had known each other for ever. We approached the last 200 metres up to the peak of the mountain on a perfect wintery day, with the whole mountain to ourselves, only a helicopter dropping off supplies to an army outpost in the far distance visible. We broke out the rope, quickdraws and ice axes and set about testing this new relationship for the first time.

We were almost 2,500 metres up in this wintery paradise and I couldn't believe she had never done anything like this before as Marie dug both feet into an almost vertical section of ice with her ice crampons, throwing an ice axe deep into the mountainside to give her some purchase to keep moving. Slowly we climbed, dragged and lifted each other, our kit and dogs up through the ice.

'I thought you were scared of heights,' I muttered to Marie at one particularly hairy bit, when we were in sight of the summit. As the final section got dangerously steep and the light was beginning to fade, we decided to tie the dogs to an iron stake hanging out from an old Second World War via ferrata line, so we could make faster progress to the top and back. We reached the final metres of chest-deep, wind-swept snow, and I got that little voice: 'You're *so* close, just keep going . . .' But it was a long way back to the truck and we didn't have much light left, so, for once, I overruled the curse and called it a day. Marie had conquered her fears with incredible determination and made it to almost 2,800 metres above sea level, on a knife-edge snowy and windy ridgeline, in the middle of the wilderness in Slovenia. We high-fived and embraced, before slithering and sliding back down to collect the dogs and then begin the steep descent.

It was then that we heard the French voice calling for help.

Truck It!

'Hold on, I'm coming,' I shouted back. I untied myself from the rope that was joining mine and Marie's harnesses in case of a fall, dug my crampons into the ice, and slowly started forcing my way back up the mountain that we had just come from. I knew immediately who it had to be. As we'd left the mountain hut in the morning, with our ice axes, crampons, spare layers and climbing rope hanging from our rucksacks, I'd looked over at the two fit French lads in their mid-twenties, rocking just trail trainers and running poles, and had assumed only serious mountaineers or lunatics would come up here with so little kit. But now, as I got closer to the source of the call, and found two lads with worried looks on their faces, wearing completely wet-through running trainers and standing in shin-deep snow, I realized I had failed to think of a third category: incompetent.

It transpired that they were Parisians visiting Slovenia for the weekend. They had also had ambitions to head to the same mountain hut we'd set our sights on, a few miles around a steep and dangerous stretch of the mountain, and they'd seen us set out up an intimidating mountain pass and thought, with two dogs in tow, it must have been doable for them, despite not having any proper winter kit. They followed us for the first couple of hours before eventually realizing they were out of their depth and returned to the steep mountain pass. Unfortunately, they'd found it was too steep and slippery to downclimb. So they were stuck. Having been in similar situations to them more times than I'd like to admit, I had no interest in telling them 'I told you so'. I approached them with a big smile and shook their hands.

'Don't worry, give me a second, let me set up this rope

and you can use it to climb down with us. We can help you round the next few dangerous sections. We don't have a spare harness so be careful, keep two hands on the rope at all times, and if you panic at any point, just shout and I'll come and get you.'

Once we'd made it back to Marie and the dogs, the next few hours we spent roping, pulling, lifting and climbing around some of the most spectacular but dangerous wintery scenery Europe had to offer. We were thousands of metres up a mountain, perched on steep ice slopes, slippery rocky sections and deep snowy chutes. The dogs had their harnesses on, so before the rescuees took their turn, I would hook them on the rope and Marie at the far end of the thirty-metre rope would whistle, and one at a time they would run, fall, slip down to her, both with huge smiles and wagging tails before unclipping and sitting patiently to heel as the two French guys would also run, fall and slip their way down. They, on the other hand, definitely didn't have big smiles or wagging tails.

A few hours later, after making it to the relative safety of a moraine field on the far side of a small valley to the other mountain hut, we shook hands, said goodbye and decided to head back to the truck. Then there was just three more hours of getting lost, abseiling the dogs down and, at one point, avoiding rockfall coming from what we think might have been a couple of the local chamois goats running high above us.

That night back at the truck, I thought about how quickly this had all become the new normal. It had only been a month since I'd set out from Wigan in the early autumn sunshine. Since then, Red and I had biked (and wagoned) our way around the sun-baked waterside at Saint-Tropez, walked, hiked and climbed our way through foothills, dived into alpine lakes, skateboarded down mountain roads and spent our days covered in snow and ice. Thirty-odd sunrises, thirty-odd sunsets. And now we had two friends along for the ride too.

I had gained a companion (and *her* protective four-legged companion) who never seemed to be negative, never seemed to find the reason not to do something. Who always said, 'Why not?' Who could see the beauty in everything you owned fitting in one blue truck. We had discovered ajvar together, the Balkan vegetable spread made from roasted peppers and tomatoes, and were now determined to eat it for most meals. There had been no grand plan. We hadn't gone the fastest or most efficient route. But I was having the time of my life.

7

Moldova the Top

'Marie, where's your knife?' I muttered as we climbed out of the truck.

'In the back by the shelves,' she whispered.

I jumped in, found the knife and tucked it into my waistband, being careful to cover it with my wintery jacket, but not so much that I couldn't get to it. Then I went outside to say hello to the six Russian men who had arrived wearing hunting gear, all of whom were about twice the size of me. We were . . . somewhere on the border between Moldova and Ukraine, a couple of miles up an unmarked track. *Bloody hell, Bobby.*

The morning had started so well. We all needed some rest and relaxation and I had decided that I'd try some fishing in the river near where we'd parked up. It had been an intense

Truck It!

four weeks since we'd left Slovenia and autumn had now very definitely become winter. In that time, we'd travelled north into Austria, where we spent a couple of nights drinking overpriced mulled wine in obscenely busy Christmas markets in Vienna. The whole city was so beautiful. Everywhere you looked there were columns, churches, palaces, arches, all glistening with gold, all crowding around each other, yet somehow it all seemed to be in harmony, especially in the lead-up to Christmas time.

It came as a shock to then cross the border into Slovakia. Tourists all but disappeared, the bright lights vanished and the roads worsened drastically. When I mentioned this on a group call with my family, my mum pointed out that we had literally just crossed the Iron Curtain into what had been the former Soviet Union. My sister, who had spent a while travelling, mocked me with: 'Bobby, you aren't even outside of Europe – just wait until you're in the middle of Uzbekistan. If Eastern Europe feels different, maybe you can't handle it and should call off the trip now.' She laughed and my mum shushed her. Bloody siblings!

Then, in a snowy field, Marie took our five-kilogram drone, travelling at twenty miles an hour, straight to the face. We had been mucking about, running around with the dogs, and as I raced towards her, where the dogs were now licking her face in concern, I had no idea what I'd find as she lay in a heap in the snow. She was giggling, which was a good sign, but her face was contorted in pain and one eye had immediately swollen shut. She had a cut beneath the eye and her lip was about four times the size it should be, too. I gently lifted her to her feet, saying, 'What did you get in the way for?' But she just narrowed her good eye and gave me *the* look. 'Too soon?' I asked.

Over the next few days, as we drove through the high Tatra mountains that run through the north of Slovakia, the temperatures plummeted and heavy snow blocked roads. So we broke out Marie's freshly purchased skiwear and went in search of some snowbound solitude.

Over the next few days, we clambered and slid up and down high, desolate mountain tracks. This kind of skiing isn't easy, and Marie found herself constantly sliding to a halt in a tangled pile of limbs and skis, both dogs jumping on her to see if she was alright as she laughed and screamed.

'Isn't this absolutely magical? How lucky are we to be doing this together . . .' Marie said.

We sat on a fallen tree and watched as thick flakes fell around us, filling up our track in the snow as if we were never there. Surrounded by spruce and Scots pine, minus ten degrees, the whole world enveloped in a heavy blanket of white, we sat in silence, lapping up every moment. The only sound was of two extremely excited dogs, bounding from one drift to another, leaping over and scrambling under fallen trees, having the time of their lives.

Back at the truck, our day-to-day had to adapt. While parked, the shower completely froze up, leaving us to brave ice-cold showers, and morning coffee and toast now required snow boots and woolly hats as we cooked and ate on our barbecue. Even so, every morning we would all burst outside into the wintery paradise with the excitement of schoolchildren at the first snowfall of the year. It was bliss.

Leaving Slovakia with our sights set on spending Christmas

in Romania, we explored a completely deserted Suchá Belá gorge, which, during the summer, is a real tourist trap. We climbed up alongside a waterfall that thickened with falling snow until we were scrambling alongside beautiful cascades of water that had partially frozen as it leapt over the edge. We drove through a landscape entirely of white, the only colour the dark green of the fir trees laden with snow, all of which was less colourful than the bruising on Marie's face, which continued to develop.

As autumn gave way to winter, we skimmed through the north of Hungary and into Romania, where we were due to meet my mum, who was on a 'cultural holiday' with some friends in central Romania. We later found out that this was code for a long weekend spent drinking exotic wine. She was heading back home for Christmas, but timings had worked for us to meet before we moved on to the coast.

'Oh my god, Marie, your face?!' my mum exclaimed as she hugged us.

'Bobby – her mouth could have nerve damage, it could be permanent.'

Marie was quiet, though I wasn't sure if it was because her face hurt, or she felt bombarded by all the questions from my mum's friends. But it was incredible to see my mum, despite the mild interrogation over wine. She said the whole family was glued to Instagram. At one point she took my hand and squeezed it: 'You've got that twinkle back in your eyes,' she said. I squeezed her hand back.

'Sorry about that,' I said to Marie later, as we got into bed, shattered from a day of socializing.

'It's all totally fine, don't worry,' she assured me. 'My face is drawing too much attention. Honestly, it looks worse than what it is. Please don't make a fuss.'

But I couldn't help mulling over the evening. I lay there, unable to sleep, turning over a throwaway comment someone had made that night: 'So, you're just on an extended holiday, then?' I had smiled, but it had rankled with me. Of course it wasn't. Was it? It had felt like I was doing more than that. Was I kidding myself that Marie and I were doing something meaningful when actually it was a glorified gap year? To make things worse, money was getting tight, there were issues with some of the sponsors and land for sale back in the UK just wasn't coming together. With the money we had left, we probably had about another month of fuel and food. But what then?

It all came to a head in Moldova a week later when I finally snapped at Rubia after she'd jumped into another field. Rubia is a Swiss shepherd. Unlike Red, who is hard-wired to retrieve sticks, swim in water and sleep, Rubia is programmed to herd, bark and scare off anything with four legs.

For the past few weeks, since joining the trip, she had been taking her job very seriously. She would drag away chairs she was tied to at coffee shops as a chihuahua, a quarter of her size, walked innocently past, scare the shit out of children leaving school as she ran towards them, go berserk at a cat sitting peacefully on a wall, or, as was the case today, jump a fence to chase after a herd of goats. In the evenings, when you'd think she would be tired and as sleepy as Red, she just went turbo-charged: growling and barking at any noise she heard outside the truck, while nominating herself as the

Truck It!

5 a.m. alarm call, pitter-pattering around and moaning for attention.

'We can't go on like this, Marie,' I said with a raised voice, dragging Rubia out of a field and away from an extremely upset pair of Moldovan farmers. We wrestled her back to the truck, apologizing to the farmers as she vigorously wagged her tail and panted, thinking she'd excelled at her mission. Marie grabbed a head torch and walked off, holding back tears.

I sat down feeling like a massive arse, and now worried about Marie, who had taken a completely unnecessary mouthful from me. About an hour later, she came back.

'Bobby,' she said, 'without Rubia, we wouldn't have ever met. I wouldn't have run up that mountain. And I know she can be hard work, but I can't abandon her.' I knew she'd already been in one relationship where the guy hadn't liked Rubia, and she wasn't prepared to make that mistake again. 'I made a commitment to look after her, so we are here as a package. It's either we both stay and we make it work, or we both leave. Imagine how overwhelming this new environment is for her. Give her some time, I know she'll settle down.'

For the first time we went to bed unsettled by our row, neither of us able to sleep. The next day we decided to delay our plans to visit the internationally unrecognized but self-declared free country of Transnistria, and instead spent a day relaxing by the Dniester river. And that's where I decided I would try my hand at fishing.

I had spent half an hour doing a vague approximation of fishing, without ever really getting near a fish, to give Marie some space to read her book a little way down the bank of the river, when a beat-up old Lada, with mismatching panels, a badly cracked windscreen and three out of four off-road tyres fitted, came bouncing down the track and parked right next to the truck.

Out climbed a big bull of a man who looked like Hagrid from Harry Potter, if he was broader and rounder. He grabbed a box and a rod out of the back of his car and then set up a fishing chair right next to where I was in a way that very much suggested this was his spot. I held my hand up and began to gather my things.

'*Sedere, sedere, sedere,*' he shouted and waved with his free hand while trying to steady the fishing rod with the other. I took that to mean 'stay' given he was pointing at the lid of his fishing box to sit on.

'Aaaah, no thank you,' I replied awkwardly, assuming his offer was for me to continue fishing next to him. 'We are heading to Transnistria.'

'Sasha,' he said, pointing at himself.

'Bobby,' I said.

'Bo-bee,' he repeated, smiling.

Marie put her book down and began to walk over to our new friend. He had a big moustache on his upper lip and the friendliest demeanour I've ever come across.

'*Da, da,*' he said as he waved me to continue reeling in, tapping his fishing box lid to sit on. I chuckled and looked at Marie, giving her the 'I'm not sure we are going anywhere fast' look.

He pulled in my line, inspected it, then shooed me off the box he'd just made me sit on, before reaching in Pandora's

Truck It!

Box, pulling out some colourful-looking hooks and passing his reel to Marie so he could attach it to my rod.

'*Daaaaaaaaaa,*' he then announced in a big, deep, proud voice as he stood, holding the rod upright in his hand like he'd just captured an enemy flag, giving it a final inspection. Then he performed a wand-like movement and cast it into the river.

My mouth dropped as he did it, having spent the morning failing to cast it beyond the shore. Marie laughed mockingly in my direction.

He turned around, grabbed his rod off Marie and cast another spell with an even bigger, more aggressive throw before sitting back down on his little fishing stool, turning and pointing to me: '*Sta.*'

For the next few hours, we sat, inspected, hummed, gestured at each other and attempted to fish.

Every now and then he would grumble, pull in his line, change his bait, and cast another spell, whipping the new bait further and further into the wide, lazy river in front.

At one point Marie asked to have a go and he spent half an hour squealing like a baby pig and laughing like a child as he tried to show her how to cast, belly-laughing when she caught the tree behind her. All three of us were in hysterics and it really didn't matter that we didn't speak a word of each other's language.

We couldn't have chosen a better way to pick our spirits up. This jolly old fisherman was just what we needed to kick us up the arse. Life's too short to hold grudges, so get over it and get on with it.

During the afternoon, one family turned up, then another,

and then another to see who we were and what we were doing. For each family that came, Sasha would pass me his rod, walk up to them with a big smile, shake their hands, then bring them down to introduce them to us. We dutifully nodded and smiled and shook hands, with no idea what anyone was saying. Some tried chatting to Marie, others stood and fished in silence.

An elderly couple and a younger girl who I assumed was their granddaughter appeared on foot later in the day. Once she had gotten over her nerves, the girl surprised us with: 'Hello, my name Natasha, I can speak little English.'

We were able to explain more about ourselves and our trip, which Natasha relayed to the group and which set our big jolly fisherman and local guide off even more. They spoke loudly, pointing at the truck, walking around and gesturing. He was now even more animated, squeaking and belly-laughing, much to the amusement of Natasha and her family.

Half an hour after saying goodbye, another Lada arrived. After spending the whole afternoon with us, Natasha and her family had come back! This time they sprung out of the car with wine, fresh chicken and a local pastry made of cabbage. Marie and I couldn't believe it.

We packed the rods away and helped set a standing table for everyone, before tucking in to a late dinner.

'We want to welcome you to Moldova. This is local food, local wine and chicken from our neighbour,' said Natasha, now growing in confidence.

I'd heard of wild travel stories before, where locals had been incredibly generous to overlanders as they passed through incredibly rural and impoverished places, but I didn't think we would get so lucky. As the sun set and darkness descended, we said our final goodbyes to the last of our visitors and retreated inside to do the washing-up.

'I can't believe how kind that was,' I said. 'Could you imagine doing that back in the south of France to a tourist?'

'Absolutely no way!' Marie laughed.

There was a moment of silence as we both thought how much better it felt than the day before. Then there was a knock at the door that made us jump and the dogs bark.

'Do you think that's Sasha?' I joked as I dried my hands and approached the door.

I switched the outside spotlights on, as by now it was pitch dark outside, to reveal two hooded men. One must have been approaching six-foot-three with a solid rugby player's frame, the other about my height (six-foot-two-and-a-half) with the wiry frame of a good amateur boxer.

'You want to drink?' said the tall guy with deep husky Russian accent, having clearly started without us.

'Errrrrrr,' I began, not quite knowing what to say to two complete strangers with their hoods up.

'My friend makes homemade wine in the village. Very good. Moldovan special wine. Come drink. You are our guests.'

Selfishly, before consulting Marie, I responded with 'Sure'. I turned to Marie, who was now drying her hands and looking at me in disbelief. 'You okay with that?' I said, turning to her as I started to fuss about the truck, then hopping down to work out the plan with my new best mates.

'We wait up there. Black car. Old. Follow us. House five minutes away.'

'No problem, give me two minutes to pack up and we will follow you.'

'Bobby, are you sure?' said a now nervous Marie as I jumped back in.

'Yeah! Look, we've met some really nice people today. I'm sure everyone's nice here. It'll be alright.' We drove, following their lights, up a winding track, quickly losing sense of where we were and which direction we were heading in. We arrived into a clearing, with the dark shape of a building off to the side. It was at that moment that the other cars arrived and four more giant shapes got out. So I went back and got the knife, gulping and praying we hadn't just walked into a trap. No one knew where we were and darkness helped to disorientate us some more.

I got out and approached the gang, standing as tall as I could, chest puffed out, putting on my best 'I'm not intimated by you guys' facial expression, but having just fully locked down the truck to make it un-stealable. I made sure I walked last through the side gate into the garden with Marie just ahead of me. In the darkness, I could just about see the shape of a low, single-storey building, with dim light spilling from behind curtains.

As we entered the rear yard, the gang made a circle and partially blocked off Marie and I as they caught up and laughed to each other. We stood awkwardly for a moment, trying to work out if it was just an innocent invitation or something more sinister.

Bang, bang . . .

The gang stopped talking and looked towards the rear wooden door of the house where the thumping noise was coming from. I braced, considered how far it was to run outside and whether it was worth running directly to the truck or momentarily trying to close the side gate to hold them up if they chased. I felt the adrenaline flooding my body. I subtly unzipped my jacket so I could get to the knife more easily without taking my eyes off the door. I felt every muscle in my body tense as . . .

Bang!

A well-dressed man, in his sixties, burst into the yard shouting, 'WELCOME TO MOLDOVA!', wielding three bottles of wine above his head in our direction. The gang cheered and started laughing. I felt my heart thudding in my chest as I laughed from utter relief. The group of hunters fussed and helped clear space on a makeshift bench, all rubbing their hands together in excitement of what was to come. I took a moment to compose myself.

'Hello, my friends, how are you? My name is Artiom, welcome to my house. Please, make yourself at home.'

We shook hands and I took note of his stylish waterproof parka jacket with the logo of a Scottish private school on, while chatter from the group picked up.

'We make all our wine ourselves here,' he said, as the glasses were filled to the brim.

'*NOROC!*' half the group shouted in harmony before downing the wine.

I turned to Marie in utter shock, who had a similar 'what is going on' look on her face.

Music was turned on, hoods were taken off, and laughter and conversations broke out.

'Wine-making is a big tradition here in Moldova,' Artiom

said in a slightly elevated voice to make himself heard above the upbeat chatter. 'Lots of people make their own wine.'

'Yes, but yours is the best, Artiom,' the big guy who met us shouted over, overhearing our conversation. 'But your wine tastes like piss compared to your schnapps.'

Upon hearing this, two of the nearest lads shouted in hoarse Russian, 'Daaaaaa schnaapppssssssss, schnapps schnapps schnapps,' which set off the others chanting.

Artiom came over all embarrassed, leaned in to us both and whispered, 'Would you like to try my schnapps? It's quite famous in the village.' As I stood back and contorted my face to communicate 'not for me thank you', Marie shouted 'Sure! Schnapps schnapps schnapps!' and joined in with the others chanting, which set everyone off laughing. I turned to her, my jaw dropping in disbelief, as she carried on chatting, only to shrug her shoulders back at me. I laughed. Clearly, I still had lots to learn about this wild travel buddy of mine.

Artiom reappeared moments later with two big, unlabelled, dirty glass bottles with clear liquid inside, to which the group cheered and downed the last of their wine only to be replaced by full glasses of the spirit. I sniffed at it warily.

'NOROC!'

We all downed it, followed by a mixture of coughs, splutters and laughs. I barely kept it down. My throat was on fire but I held my thumb up. 'Very good,' I spluttered politely.

Over the next half an hour, home-grown apples, nuts and assorted alcoholic beverages were brought out before everyone started to look noticeably more pissed.

'Please take this as a gift from Moldova,' Artiom said, handing me a plastic water bottle filled with a red liquid,

Truck It!

using both hands, like he was gifting a royal family member a sword. 'This is my favourite sweet red wine. It is very good. Just make sure you buy Moldovan wine when you can. It is the best in the world,' he added, raising his voice at the end, which set off another cheer.

He laughed, and we finished off our glasses and slowly walked out of the garden to the front, where the truck was still thankfully parked.

I felt the knife in my pocket and felt suddenly ashamed. How could I have thought they had anything but good intentions?

Just before we left, the first big guy we had met, who I now knew was called Cornel, said: 'My brother Vasile and I would like to invite you for dinner at my house. It is five minutes away. Nikita my wife speaks good English and makes a very good, pickled cabbage soup. Please. It would be my honour.'

We agreed, then shook hands with the other drunken members of the crew as they each got into a jeep, a Lada and a police car before driving off.

Fifteen extremely carefully driven minutes later, we arrived at a narrow dirt street. Vasile leaned out of the window of his car as we passed a house and waved vigorously, indicating that this was their home.

We carried on to the top of the street and onto a ploughed field, which happened to be a viewpoint. 'That's Ukraine . . . that's the school I teach at . . . that's where we met you,' Cornil pointed out as we stood looking out at the dark landscape, drinking whiskey to keep our stomachs warm from the biting cold wind.

'Okay, now come. Dinner is ready.'

We left the truck on the ploughed field and marched down the track, through metal gates and into a partially built, half-finished home.

A woman, Nakita, was busy fussing at the kitchen as we entered and said hello, as two children ran across the room in their pyjamas to give Vasile a big hug.

'I hope my brother and my husband have been behaving themselves,' Nakita said inquisitively with a smile on her face as we hugged hello.

'Yes, we have,' Cornil assured her. 'We took Boddy and Mary to see Artiom' – which got him a side-eyed look of disapproval back from his well-spoken sister stood stirring the soup.

'It was all good, don't worry,' he said, before turning to us and winking, then pointing for us to sit down.

For the rest of the evening, we chatted to what turned out to be the most wholesome, kind and generous young family I'd ever met. Cornil lived down the street but ate with us, despite swaying in his chair vigorously a number of times, while Vasil silently threw down as much bread as his small frame could handle.

'We don't have much money here in Moldova,' said Vasil. 'But we are happy and we are kind.'

'I go to drive in England for Amazon next month,' said Vasil, with a mouthful of yet more bread, much to my surprise and the obvious disapproval of his wife, who swung the dishcloth at him. 'We can earn more money in three months driving in Birg-ming-Ham than we can in a year here in Moldova. I leave in two weeks.'

Truck It!

I thought of the warmth and happiness there was here, of leaving it all to travel away from your family and friends. My dad had worked as a lorry driver his whole life, so I had some understanding of it, but the idea of Vasil being away for three months at a time from the family he clearly adored left me contemplating life here versus back in the UK.

As the evening came to an end, we hugged goodbye and walked out the door with Cornil leading the way, walking as if he was on a boat on a stormy sea.

'I must go sleep. I lecture at university in the morning,' he slurred, giving each of us a big bear hug, nestling his head into the top of ours before stumbling off down the dark street.

We walked back up to the truck, exhausted but full of love for the world.

We lay thinking about what had happened, about the kindness of strangers willing to share whatever they had with us. I didn't know if it was the vast amounts of wine and spirits, but I was feeling quite emotional about how lucky we were to have seen that kind of pure generosity. The past year had really hammered home how important family was to me. I had spent so long away from mine when I'd been living down south, but owed them so much for their support in the most difficult of times. I reached for my phone and sent my mum a text message telling her I loved her, then sent one to my dad telling him I'd caught a massive fish.

'*NOROC!*' Marie shouted, lifting her hand in front of her. We laughed, kissed, turned the lights off and fell asleep to the sound of the wind in the trees.

8

Romanic

The Romanian truck driver was glaring at me in a way that made it clear he would very much like to punch me. He was shouting and gesturing up at the truck using words that I was almost certain weren't terms of endearment. He continued to scream and swear at the top of his voice, squaring up to me so I could feel his breath on my skin, pointing back at the miles and miles of queuing trucks we had just driven past. It was mid-December on the border between Moldova and Romania, and things were getting a bit spicy.

'I'm not a bloody lorry,' I swore back at him, as the uninterested border guard watched us both and leaned back in his chair to call the boss. 'I'm a truck.'

It had been much easier a couple of days before when we'd nipped over the 'border' into Transnistria for twelve hours. Depending on how you look at it this thin strip of land in between the Dniester river and Ukraine is either a separatist region, having broken away from Moldova and self-declared as a state, supported by Russia. Or, according to our Moldovan friend, Cornil, as he rooted around for more spirits: 'It's Moldova!'

The day we turned up to the imaginary border, we were greeted by a dozen soldiers wearing Russian uniform, sat smoking on a Russian tank, which we had to drive around as it was blocking the road to slow traffic.

For the first time, I took a big gulp, wondering if we'd made a bad call.

No passports were stamped, no official visa issued. They wrote down our passport details in a dusty handwritten ledger, before passing over something that looked like a fairground-ride ticket.

'Twelve hours,' said the woman – who let's just say I wouldn't have wanted to meet in a dark alley late at night – in a thick Russian accent.

We went to the 'capital', which resembled Bolton on an okay day, populated by grey, sad-looking people. It was unnervingly empty for such a big place, which gave it an eerie feel.

Busses ran on overhead power cables and looked like something from the sixties, while the buildings were caught in a time warp from the Soviet era, all imposing boxes of concrete with patriotic statues and murals.

We attempted to pay for coffee but all our cards and cash were declined. In a moment of unexpected generosity, a girl who was learning English from her father, who worked in 'IT overseas' (AKA A RUSSIAN SPY), paid for us.

'I have never seen a tourist here. How did you come here?' the young girl asked. After telling her our story, she looked bewildered: 'It is not possible, no.' We laughed and replied something along the lines of, 'Yeah we don't know what we are doing here either' followed by a nervous giggle.

We timidly walked around for another hour or so, barely speaking a word to each other while all the inquisitive locals gawped at us.

'Let's get out of here,' I whispered, and began praying none of the few hundred soldiers and military personnel we passed would take issue with our presence as we came bouncing past.

But right now, stood on the periphery of the very real Moldova–Romania border, with the compass set back southwest towards the Balkans, I found myself longing for an imaginary one. Bearing in mind that this is a border where the European Union technically ends and non-EU begins, it is a border that takes itself very seriously. Now, if you've never crossed a border like this, I want you to imagine a badly built, then poorly maintained British industrial estate from the 1980s. Now just keep building new buildings every decade or so, but don't demolish the old ones – just partly abandon them and make sure the new areas don't connect with the old in any logical manner. Have vehicles mount curbs and ignore any sort of sense of order as they pass through. Now remove any sort of helpful signage, just a few faded ones – some on the old buildings, some on the new ones, to confuse anyone passing through.

Now, rather than an orderly queue of vehicles trying to cross, add in a few thousand lorries and get them all to form

Truck It!

twelve or so terrible queues, and then rugby-scrum them into a single lane for processing over the course of around thirty-six hours of inching forward. For good measure, throw in a few stray dogs as well as thirty or so vehicles that have broken down, been abandoned or partly stripped to help disrupt any orderly queue that has accidentally formed.

Toilets? Nope. Fill what bushes remain in this urban nightmare with toilet paper and human excrement. Now, to top it all off, add one extremely angry truck driver, almost certainly with chronic haemorrhoids, who thinks me and Marie are trying to push into the queue.

We'd already been trying for hours by the time he arrived on the scene. As we crawled along with a dull grey December sky above, it felt a very long way from the beginning of our trip two months before and the clear blue skies of France. When we'd first arrived at the border, we'd attempted to drive through the tourist/car/coach portal of the border, but immediately got waved away by the guard. 'No car,' he said.

I shrugged, saying, 'Well, I guess we'll try with the trucks then,' as we went the wrong way up a one-way lane and skipped to the front of the truck queue, blocking any of the drivers moving. And that's where we'd been accosted by my new best mate.

'Wait,' shouted the border guard as the driver stormed off to rally more support from the now growing number of annoyed-looking drivers who were lingering outside their trucks, all staring daggers at us in their flip-flops.

'Okay, you go with trucks. But wait. We cannot let you through now. The drivers are not happy.' So, apparently as a token gesture, we waited twenty minutes as my old mucker got back in his lorry and drove through. Marie and I both kept our heads down. I wasn't sure if it was still that comment of 'extended holiday' echoing in my head from Romania, but something about this process was really winding me up. It was as if there was no place for what we were doing. This border crossing was the physical representation of the strangeness of our trip: were we just on holiday? Was this a lorry or a truck? There was no place for us.

'Okay, you go now,' shouted the guard.

'Where?' I responded, holding my hand up in a shrug.

A silent aggressive hand gesture in the general direction of the border was his response.

We joined another queue and inched forward, accepting utter defeat until a couple of hours later a helpful lorry driver waved at us to follow him.

'What a nice guy, Marie, look.'

We set off following him through what looked like a special lane for, well, we weren't actually too sure, but as we started to bypass a long queue of lorries all fighting for space, I had just started to smile when a border guard jumped out to stop us as our helpful escort disappeared into the distance.

'Sorry, we don't know where to go, no one is telling us,' said Marie to the guard, whose job you couldn't pay me enough money to do.

'What are you doing here? You need to be with the coaches.'

I laughed.

'We were told to come this way at the gate. We're not a coach.'

'No. Go back.' His tone was forceful as if he held authority.

'Coaches.' There was no debate.

Truck It!

I let out a big sigh as Marie cursed in French.

I mounted a curb three times to turn around as we slowly picked our way back through oncoming traffic before turning into the coach queue.

'What are you doing here?' It was another guard, looking equally annoyed at us.

'You have got to be kidding me.'

'You cross with the trucks.'

I jumped out. 'I'm sorry, no, we started with cars, then went to trucks, then crossed the other way with the coaches, we came in with the trucks, we got refused, we are now here and now we are getting refused again.'

'No English. Trucks.'

I thought my head was actually going to explode. Maybe this would be it. The entire rest of the trip would be joining queues and being told to start again. Marie and I would grow old here, just moving from queue to queue. To cap it all, I was starving. I'd eaten as many of the stuffed polenta balls that were my favourite Romanian food as I could at a stall on the way to the border, but we had arrived at about midday. It was now getting dark. I wouldn't even have turned my nose up at the dry-cured bear we'd eaten by accident the other day. There were no more than two lights working in a row across this massive industrial estate, leaving big areas of darkness full of weird shadows scurrying around.

However, in a gesture born of either sympathy or impatience, the border guard walked round a derelict toilet block building, which was still piling up with fresh excrement, and opened a gate to bypass the majority of the truck queue we'd just driven past.

We forced our way into the pack of trucks, ten or so back from what we now assumed was the front of the line, but we really had no idea. That night we must have pissed off half of the Moldovan truck-driving community.

It was approaching 9 p.m. as we edged near the front of the queue, which had begun to turn into a frenzy. Truck drivers in their socks and flip-flops ran back and forth towards a small open-sided warehouse building, before running back in a fluster and setting off as if being chased by an army, leaning on their horns for minutes until any driver who was blocking their exit ran back to their vehicle and floored it as well.

'Marie, I'm having an identity crisis here,' I shouted. 'What are we?'

We didn't have a clue what was going on, or where we were, or where we were supposed to go. Nor did any of the border guards for that matter.

We stopped vaguely near the warehouse, but certainly not alongside, hopped out and headed towards a scrummage of people to work out what we needed to do to escape this trucking hell.

'OIIIIIIII BLABALBALBALAAALA,' a guard shouted, waving something at me, to which I came across all British with, 'I'm terribly sorry, I've not a clue what I'm doing.'

He shouted again, waving at me vigorously, which set the rest of the clowns hanging around wearing border guards outfits into fits of laughter.

After he got bored and moved on to another driver, I went in search of the next steps.

'WHAT YOU DO? NO. There.'

Truck It!

He pointed to a badly signposted, badly lit portacabin, twenty metres away, just outside the warehouse. 'Police stamp first,' he shouted from inside his box marked 'customs'.

Like a lost child in the worst zoo ever, I walk towards the cabin and gave a polite knock and waited a moment to enter before a rotund Romanian driver, wearing flip-flops, shorts from his young teenage daughter and an off-white vest, burst swearing out of the door, followed by the border guard, who was walking after him waving and swearing.

'Is this police stamp?' I nervously said as they both stopped swearing at each other.

He waved me in, took zero time to inspect both our passports, ignored the fact Marie wasn't present, stamped them and waved me outside. Approaching the customs box, which was the size of two British telephone boxes, despite being the main processing centre for what must have been thousands of drivers, a fight broke out. I literally stood there in complete shock. There was a group of twenty-five, maybe thirty, tired and pissed-off-looking drivers trying to push their way to the front of the customs box, and two or three towards the back were now throwing punches and grappling.

I turned in the direction of the truck to see if Marie was watching this pantomime play out. The border guards took no action bar a token shout over the crowd, which was ignored. None of the other official clowns even moved an inch or looked up from scrolling on their phones.

I took my chance and leaned in and passed our passports and car documents to the one official who had now bothered to look up.

In the midst of this war zone was, however, one very busy

guy wearing camo and carrying a ladder. He seemed to be the sole inspector for every truck trying to pass through, as he was the only one in sight doing any work.

He was up and down a ladder quicker than any busy London window cleaner, doing a relatively thorough job as the rest of his group did exactly nothing.

There was suddenly a loud whistle, which caught the attention of half of the group who weren't fighting on the floor. Camo guy was pointing with a long straight arm at the truck, and to Rubia, whose head was sticking out of the window, having heard the ruckus and gone to investigate.

'DOG. NO DOG. PASSPORT,' he shouted over to me.

I stuck out like a sore thumb among the agitated, badly dressed Eastern European drivers. He looked right at me in the crowd and pointed to me, then Rubia.

Shit.

I walked over to the man who continued to shout 'DOG PASSPORT' at me, pointing at the dog, even when he was only about a metre away from my face.

I nodded in agreement, feeling completely overwhelmed by what was going on.

I opened the door and Marie passed the two EU passports for the dogs. Red's we'd managed to secure by using the extended family member's address to register him as a French dog, during the first down days of the trip.

He opened a few random pages, which got him scowling. 'DATE?!' he bellowed at me, still stood within whispering distance.

'Errrr . . .'

'DATE,' he shouted again, which made me lean back to

Truck It!

avoid being deafened. I went to open to the correct page and pointed to a random vet stamp, not knowing what he was actually asking.

'2025,' I said as a gamble.

He slapped the passport shut and threw it into my chest.

'DATTTEE,' he said, opening the second passport as I repeated the same response.

After throwing the second dog passport back to me, he then walked off, having completely lost interest.

I turned to look up to Marie, who was open-mouthed as I gave a shrug as if to say, 'I have no idea what's going on.'

'GREAT BRITANNIA! GREAT BRITANNIA!' shouted the border guard, leaning his torso out of his booth. The huddle of men had now calmed down and one driver was being held back from pummelling a much younger, more athletic driver.

I couldn't get to the booth despite the guard shouting and waving to make way. Instead, he tossed each passport one by one into the crowd towards me, which had the truck documents tucked in.

I walked back to the truck, jumped in and looked around.

'Are we done? No one's actually checked the truck, have they?' I said.

'Just drive,' said Marie.

I started the truck up and set off tentatively, expecting to hear a shout or whistle. Nothing came.

We went round a few more buildings, wrongly marked roundabouts and a truck having its tyre changed.

'Is that it? Are we back in the EU?' I said, as Marie scowled out of the window trying to figure out where we were. 'Marie, if that's how all commercial trade gets in and out of the

European Union, then it's a complete joke! That was an absolute shit show!' I said, still slightly shaken from the twelve-hour ordeal.

'Just drive,' said Marie, laughing.

We turned back to the dogs in their bed, who looked like they were just waking up from a long relaxing nap, having missed the entire day. 'Right, where are we going next?' I asked.

Marie shrugged.

'The sea?'

'Yeah, alright,' she responded.

I pulled out my phone, stuck a pin on the nearest patch of blue and off we went.

9

Resolutions in Romania

Everyone has their Christmas traditions. My new one is that every year I want to go skinny-dipping on a deserted Romanian beach, then sit and drink and laugh and watch the sunset light the clouds on fire.

We had been woken up at seven that morning by a knock on the door, and I assumed it was the police come to move us on. We were on Plaja Vadu, a stretch of coast completely deserted in winter, probably thanks to the miles of flooded tracks we had to navigate. We'd gone there after the pin I'd dropped into the blue turned out to be the Danube Delta, home to some of the most diverse wildlife in all of Europe in summer. In the winter, however, it was playing host to three half-drunk Romanian men, ten burnt-out cars and a couple of extremely noisy woodpigeons. We left before depression took hold.

Bobby Bolton

When I heard the knock at the door, I was already imagining what the police officer who goes patrolling the beach on Christmas Eve is like.

'Pass me the bribe money?' I asked Marie as I hastily got changed and got the dogs under control.

I opened the door to a good-looking twenty-year-old guy with bed hair and tired-looking eyes. 'Hello, I'm so sorry, can you help me? We are stuck and no one is around.'

I looked out to the far end of the beach, which was a good mile or so away, to see the rough outline of a white car with its nose pitched down towards the sand.

'Yeah, no problem,' I said, jumping out and up onto the roof. 'Take these recovery boards and this shovel and give me ten minutes and I'll follow you up there.'

It turned out Alex was on a first date and, presumably keen to make a good impression, had driven his lady friend two hours from Bucharest in his Vauxhall Corsa to watch the sunset. Unfortunately, they'd got snagged in the sand and he'd had to spend a sleepless cold night sat alongside his date, who thought she was being taken to a nice restaurant for the evening. As the sun came up, they'd seen the truck, then left it as long as they could before coming and asking for help. As the dogs ran up and down the beach, Alex, Marie and I dug the car out, while his date gave the distinct impression that this wasn't what she had been expecting.

'I wonder what she thought of that date?' smiled Marie as they eventually drove off.

'I'd have said yes to a second date to him,' she said cheekily, which made me giggle.

Truck It!

It made me grateful, yet again, that Marie saw the world the way she did. I knew that if exactly the same thing had happened to us, then she'd have been making the best and laughing about it.

As Europeans are accustomed to celebrating on Christmas Eve rather than the twenty-fifth, later that evening we exchanged the petrol station Christmas presents we'd bought each other and drank until we ran into the icy cold sea naked, shrieking and laughing. The dogs looked at us with parental concern, definitely not joining in.

And despite the presents handed over being wrapped in tin foil, and despite being absent from our families at my favourite time of the year, it was a perfect day. We had childish fun playing cricket with the shovel, building a little fire and watching the sun set from the roof of the cab.

On Christmas morning, feeling slightly delicate from too much cheap Moldovan wine, we drove into the city of Constanta, a busy port city with restaurants and nightclubs, dotted with beautiful ruins. It turned out to be one of the oldest cities in the whole of Europe, having been settled almost 600 years before London.

We were immediately called into action once again when an old-school Russian sailor gave us proper Russian vodka and some fuel money in thanks for digging his car free from the beach. I was still too hungover to look at it and hid it in a cupboard. I called both my mum and my dad, wished them a happy Christmas. It was strange to think about them, about to have the classic family Christmas, and me, with sand from the Black Sea still in my ears. Christmas was definitely one of those times it was brought home just how far away we were, and this was the first time I'd been so far away for the festive period.

We were just beginning to think about where to head next when a message popped up on my phone:

Bobby it is Alex from the beach. I want to invite you to horse ride with me. Let's meet in three days. Oh and the girl didn't want to go on a second date lol.

So, a few days later, after a brief stop at a ski resort for the morning, we dashed to some stables to meet Alex for an afternoon's ride.

'What's your riding ability?' said a very well-to-do instructor wearing all the right gear, looking fantastic.

'Very good,' I responded confidently, having never ridden a horse before.

'Okay then. This is your horse. His name is Ferrari.'

'Why did you call him Ferrari?'

'I'm sure you will find out,' the nice lady said, passing me the reins with a smile, probably seeing through my white lie as I stood there in builders' steel-toe-capped boots.

Thirty minutes later, I found myself grabbing some of Ferrari's mane with one hand and the saddle with the other as the group of excellent riders, Marie included, set off at full pelt. My first thought was, *I wish I'd worn tighter underwear.* The second was that I might die, closely followed by wishing I'd been given a horse called Nissan Micra.

Taking me at my word, no one had told me anything about how to ride a horse. I was bucked, thrown and slammed around as Ferrari shot off with no direction from me. He had seen his mates set off with their riders screaming words of encouragement and clearly fancied a slice of the action.

Truck It!

Marie found it absolutely hilarious as she turned around at full gallop and used her phone to record me holding on for dear life as we sped down the icy track.

After what felt like an hour, we slowed down and I tried to recover some composure and salvage what remained of my testicles. Marie turned and navigated her way over serenely, crying with laughter. Alex arrived just in time to hear me whimper, 'Well, I don't think we'll ever be able to have kids.'

Alex proudly offered us a special cigarette, which I declined. I didn't need anything that might impede my skills further. Alex was clearly a really nice young guy, full of enthusiasm and the desire for adventure and love for his country. But he also had a slightly dangerous glint in his eye that I recognized. He had a touch of the crazy about him. Finally, after two hours, I was able to dismount, wincing down from Ferrari, who I swear smiled at me. Then Alex took Marie and me halfway up a mountain in the pitch dark to visit a cave monastery he'd heard about, only to be attacked by four mountain guardian dogs, owned by a wild-looking priest who drove a modified Suzuki Samari jeep with mud terrain tyres, a six-inch lift, snorkel and winch. Very much my kind of priest!

Red was giving it back as good as he got, which I was extremely proud of, but I had to get stuck in twice with a big stick to keep the wolf dogs from tearing his limbs off.

By this point, Alex had smoked several 'cigarettes' and wanted to climb to the summit of the mountain in the dark. Wishing him the very best of luck, we made our excuses and headed back down to the truck.

As a final stop in Romania, we drove 300-odd miles west towards Sibiu, where we were planning to spend New Year's Eve. On the way, we decided to cross the Transfagarasan highway, which Jeremy Clarkson had once coined 'the best driving road in the world', but we arrived to find deep snow drifts and 'road closed' signs.

'Oh well, tomorrow let's head up that cable car and see if we can summit another peak with the mountaineering kit,' I said, trying to salvage something from the effort of driving all the way there.

Early the next morning, we took the first cable car to the top, where we were unexpectedly greeted with man-made igloos selling mulled wine, kids running off to play with toboggans, and a mountain lodge offering overnight digs to tourists who were skidding about in trainers on the ice.

After throwing on our winter climbing kit, we convinced the reluctant dogs to follow us up yet another snowy mountain. In bright sunlight, we climbed until we were above the cloud. We scaled ridges until we were on top of the world, in a scene of white and blue, with the cleanest, coldest mountain air stinging our lungs. At one point we bumped into a guy who shouted, 'Welcome to Romania!' and offered us a slug of yet another unknown alcoholic drink from his hip flask. 'NOROC!'

At one point, my shadow was cast against the mountain hundreds of metres below, supersized and surrounded by a rainbow halo in what is known as a Brocken spectre. I stood with my arms stretched outside, looking up to the heavens.

'MARIE! LOOK! BEHOLD! I AM A MESSENGER FROM GOD!' I shouted. I turned back towards her as she didn't say anything, only to receive a snowball in the face as she brought me back down to earth.

At the summit, we looked down and just smiled from the joy of where we were, roped together, panting from the exertion.

On the way back down, I decided we should take a shortcut down a steep section of the mountain. It was going to save us retracing our steps back along a snowy ridgeline, but it was too steep to walk, so I suggested we slide down, using our ice axes to control the speed.

I sat down, set off and shouted back instructions as I demonstrated how to keep your feet up so your spikes don't get caught and digging in the ice axe behind you with both hands to one side like a paddle in a canoe.

'Okay, your turn,' I said, calling up to Marie, who was now twenty metres or so up the steep snowy slope. She set off slowly, making a running motion with her feet to get going. But as she slid past me, I realized she was struggling to stay in control. 'Dig the axe in deeper to slow down!' I called, but I watched as her speed increased from a jog, to a sprint, to fully out of control. Then her feet spikes dug in the snow as she struggled to keep them in the air. It immediately sent her into a fast topple, side to side and head over heels, over and over and over again, picking up speed all the time. I lost sight of her as she went over the brow of something, I couldn't tell what. A gentle hillock, or a cliff? *She could be dead*, I thought. The dogs set off like rockets down after her.

I'd had the drone in the air to film what I thought was going to be a fun moment and I looked down at the screen to see her tumbling down towards a section of the mountain where the snow gave way to lumps of rocks poking through. I suddenly couldn't remember if she had her helmet on. 'Shit!' I exclaimed. I threw my bag back on and slid the 200 metres down to where she was and arrived to find her holding her knee, gritting her teeth as the dogs were once again trying to lick her. This time she wasn't batting them away.

I couldn't believe it. Her face was only just recovering from the drone incident.

'Marie! Are you okay?'

She started to cry, lying there, not saying a word.

I looked up and saw she had come to a stop at the beginning of a boulder field. If she'd gone tumbling into that, who knows what could have happened. I couldn't bear to think.

'Holy shit, you've been lucky,' I said.

I helped her sit upright, where she took a big deep breath and attempted to move her leg.

'Is it broken?' I asked. She responded with a shake of the head. 'Can you stand?'

'*Attendez* one minute, please?' she whispered back.

I had no idea what to do. We were a long hike away from the gondola, and I doubt mountain rescue existed in this part of the world. Whatever was going to play out, it was going to be hard work.

'Okay, I'm ready.' She held out her hands so I could help her stand.

She limped to a stand and took two painfully laboured steps forward, before putting both hands on her good leg.

'It's my knee. It hurts like hell, but it will be okay. We'd better go before we get trapped up here.'

She shook off my offers of help and began limping down

through the boulder field, using her ice axe as a small walking stick, before we had to tackle going up and over a mountain pass.

I knew Marie was tough, but I hadn't realized how tough until that walk. For two hours, she limped in silence, with tears in her eyes, refusing any help, stopping every now and then to gather her strength.

'I think we'll take a little break from mountains,' I said as we sat in the cable car.

We welcomed in the new year dancing (Marie limping) with a couple of thousand locals to a band dressed in wolf and bear skins, accompanied by what looked like six milk maids in traditional Swiss costume.

As midnight came, we kissed as the fireworks erupted.

'I'm so lucky,' I whispered in her ear.

'Me too,' she said back as we embraced in a beautifully long hug surrounded by thousands of strangers.

2023 had been one hell of a year. I'd been at the lowest point in my life, broke, living in a caravan. And yet a drunken idea to drive to the far side of the world had been the fuel to set me off on a life-changing trip. I was only three months in and I'd seen and done more in that time than I would have done in a decade back in my old life.

If next year was going to be just as incredible, I – no, *we* – were going to have one hell of a story to tell when we got home. Bring it on!

10

Montenegro M G

'Dad, I think we're actually screwed this time.'

My voice was calm but only just.

'Where are you?' he asked.

I looked around me. All I could see was trees, rocks and snow.

'Literally the middle of nowhere,' I said.

This wasn't an exaggeration. It was late January and we were in the Durmitor National Park in Montenegro, high in the Dinaric Alps, several hours' drive from anything resembling a proper road.

We had spent the previous month heading back around 600 miles west, through the north of Serbia and into Croatia. (I never said we were taking the quick route!) Pausing only briefly to rescue a toothless farmer's truck from the mud and toast ourselves with a clear liquid, which we swigged before shouting 'Schnapps!', our plan was to turn left when he hit the coast.

At the Plitvice Lakes National Park, we walked through a landscape of snow, trees and water so stripped of colour it felt like being in a black-and-white photograph. Red streaking through the white was the most colourful thing there. We travelled south down the eastern coast of the Adriatic in the region known as Dalmatia. I explained to Red that this area was known for some very famous dogs, but he was completely unimpressed. The sun came out and we zigzagged from island to island, along empty roads and tracks, parking up next to forgotten beaches and diving into deserted coves. It was as if someone had turned the colour back on, the deep green of the bushes, the blue of the sky and water and the pale stone darkening from the sea. The sun set in pale pinks and oranges.

'Do you fancy popping into Bosnia?' I had said while we sat watching a guy catch octopus with his bare hands near Split.

'Sure, what's there?' asked Marie.

'I'm not sure. Why don't we go see?'

Ten days later, and we were still there. We'd driven past the one-hundred-foot-tall cross overlooking Old Mostar. From the top of the hill we looked down at the jumble of red-tile roofs, nestling among the hills. We enjoyed a day ambling round the old town, visiting the war museum, before once again getting lost and stumbling quite literally into the grounds surrounding Tito's £20 billion nuclear war bunker, built in the fifties during the Cold War. Then we wound our way east through high mountain roads, stopping to ski our way past frozen waterfalls into spiked icicles. At Trnovo, the dogs dragged us through beech trees as we ski-trekked through a deserted forest. I had grown up in an era where you hear the word Bosnia and you think of war, but it was such an incredible place, with the most beautiful natural landscapes and historical cities to explore.

Approaching Montenegro, we drove over an incredible bridge high over a mountain valley and through tunnels covered with a ceiling of huge icicles. Under a bare hut, we looked down over the valley spread far below us. At first, the half-metre flurries of snow that fell out of the sky were amazing, as we'd been skiing our way around this tiny mountainous country on the Balkan peninsula, nestled in between Bosnia to the north and Albania to the south. In bright sun, with blue skies, we'd spend the whole day mucking about in fresh powder, laughing with pure joy. Then the fuel line froze. It was -15 and suddenly the air was thick with snow and the remote location, surrounded by dark pine trees, started to seem a bit less magical. Skinny-dipping in the Black Sea seemed like a very long time ago.

That first night, as the diesel night heater stopped working, I was thankful for the insulation I'd fitted, as it kept us warm enough that we had to crack a window open. In the morning, with classic Bobby enthusiasm, I attempted to start the truck, pumping and priming the fuel lines to try to force it into life, despite a quick inspection showing the fuel was frozen into a sort of gel.

'If I can just get it going enough to bring a little warmth to the engine, it should melt the fuel,' I explained to Marie,

Truck It!

who stood nervously looking over my shoulder the next day.

I didn't admit fully to my colossal cock-up half an hour later when I realized I had flattened the batteries trying to force it to start. We took the dogs for a walk to take our minds off things, then after Marie had set off back to the truck, I sneakily called my dad.

'I'm serious. My only hope is that the tank warms up somehow in the sun. But it's cloudy.' My dad, practical as ever, said, if it came to it, we should gather twigs and make a very controlled, very careful fire under the fuel tank. He also said that we might be able to connect the jump leads to our auxiliary batteries and use that to start the engine once the fuel was liquid again.

'But make sure you turn everything in the truck off,' he warned, 'you need to conserve battery.'

I didn't tell him that we'd snapped a solar panel lead and currently only had drained the batteries dangerously low to 18 per cent. I paused at the top of a hill in the snow as the light began to fade, biting my nails. We were so blanketed in snow that even our tracks had been covered over. And no one without some serious four-wheel drive was getting up here in this weather to help us. Our engine battery was flat, our auxiliary batteries running out, our solar power broken. The last thing my dad said to me was, 'Whatever happens, you'll figure it out.'

Not for the first time, I was grateful I came from a long line of figurer-outers. My dad's dad, Norman, had run his own business and when I asked what had made it successful, my dad said it was down to hard work and his ability to work out how to fix pretty much anything. He was entirely self-taught, had left school as soon as he was allowed and had severe dyslexia, but he devised his own system for counting, using shapes he drew, so he could run his business. He was always tinkering with something. He had one of those brains that just liked to solve problems, whether it was driving in a forklift an employee's wife who was too drunk to stand home, or dismantling an old Honda motorbike and turning it into a full car-sized go-cart, complete with a fabricated pedal system for the throttle, so I could learn how to use them when I was fourteen.

My dad was driving from the time he could reach the pedals as well. It was his job to move the trailers around the yard with a truck. Once, when he was fourteen, he was left to queue for petrol on a hill, while Norman went to do a job. The brakes of the coal truck in front gave out and it careered backwards, smashing the windscreen and half burying my dad. Norman was swiftly summoned and dug his screaming young adolescent son out of the cab, before setting him down outside the truck to pull himself together, while Norman went to have 'a word' with the driver of the coal truck.

Another time, he bought a fire-damaged car and worked on it to get it road-worthy. On the first test run, he was pulled over by the police for speeding, at which point he was quick to declare that the car had been in a fire and the instrument panel had suffered smoke damage, rendering the speedometer unreadable. All that could be seen was the red hand moving around. 'Sorry, sir.'

Norman managed to talk the police officer into tailing Norman and flashing his lights at certain speeds, at which

Truck It!

point, using Irene's lip stick, he would mark the speed on the dashboard.

My dad had absorbed that 'just get on with it' worldview and that was how he'd raised me. One of my strongest memories is sitting in my dad's pickup, barely able to reach the pedals as he towed it in his truck. On speakerphone, my dad talked me through narrow country lanes: 'Slow down . . . brake brake brake . . . okay, keep in line with me,' he repeated over and over again as I steered his pride and joy, ten feet behind. We arrived and I almost cried with relief. But this, and a hundred other times like it, meant that I always believed I'd get myself out of any scrape.

I made the decision not to tell Marie quite how up against it we were with flat batteries and frozen fuel, quietly unplugging the fridge when we returned to the truck. I looked up the weather forecast. It ranged between minus one and minus eleven.

'It's now or never,' I said. I took Marie's hairdryer, cut the lead in half, badly wired a 5-metre extension piece in the middle from an offcut I had as spare, and asked her to lie underneath to thaw out the fuel filter.

'The sun has warmed the tank and fuel enough, I think, but the filter and lines look frozen, so attack those with the hairdryer, please,' I asked as I passed the hairdryer to Marie, who lay in the snow under the truck.

For the next hour as the last of the sun's energy faded, Marie hair-dried while I pumped, fettled and kept an eye on the battery level.

'That'll do,' I shouted. 'Seven per cent power left. I hope that's enough.'

Grabbing my dad's prized possessions that he'd lent me for the trip, I attached one end to the dead truck batteries and the other to the 7 per cent charged auxiliary batteries, and hopped in.

I had been too nervous to film all day. As I turned the key, the truck coughed and spluttered and failed to start. I tried again: 'Come oooooooon!' Again it spluttered and then, finally, after what seemed like hours, came to life, letting out a big puff of white smoke from the exhaust that rose in a big fluffy ball in the still air.

Marie and I screamed 'wahoooooo!' in unison. I sat for a few minutes in the cab, feathering the throttle to make sure she didn't die, while Marie hastily packed everything up and threw it inside.

With absolutely zero regard for the condition of the steep snowy track heading back down the mountain, I engaged full angry off-road mode and ploughed our way through the deep snow.

Ice, especially wet ice after a day of sun, is far more slippery than fresh snow, which, if not compacted, actually gives you a lot of traction.

With desperation still at my fingertips, we made it down the mountain to the nearest fuel station, where we put in the most expensive winter-grade anti-freezing diesel, buying a few handfuls of emergency defrosting additives as well, just in case we got caught out again. After we handed over an eye-watering amount of cash, we both laughed with relief.

We drove down out of the mountains and camped on the shore of the massive Lake Skadar, the largest in southern Europe, which straddles Montenegro and Albania. A hundred

Truck It!

kilometres south, and it was like we were in a different world. As we watched the dogs swimming in the lake, we both exhaled a deep breath. It hadn't always been totally smooth sailing, but Marie and I had made it through this first part of the trip. Max had been partly right: moving in with someone at the same time as travelling around the world had been intense, but we had totally got into the swing of it. And now I genuinely couldn't imagine my life without Marie and Rubia. Who would suddenly appear with one of her miracle crêpes? Who would I sing at the top of my lungs to as I drove? Who would I share the sunsets with?

As January turned into February and we pointed the truck south and east, it felt as if we were leaving the deep winter behind.

11

Istanbullish

'Oi!'

I shouted at the young skinny Turkish guy who had hold of both the dogs' leads, yanking them by the neck. Marie watched on with wide eyes. A few minutes earlier, we had been standing in the car park where we'd parked the truck when he'd walked past the truck in the opposite direction, and Red, in an uncharacteristic moment, had started barking, staring straight at him. I walked over to him now with my palms outstretched as he refused to let Red and Rubia go.

'Listen, what's going on, fella?'

He responded, irate, narrowing his eyes, and gave the dogs two painful-looking tugs again. Both of them stood wide-eyed, wondering what the hell was going on, looking at me in terror.

Truck It!

I pulled my phone out, opened Google Translate and hit Turkish.

'Here, type, Turkish. Translate, English,' I said, as if talking to a child while miming to release the dogs.

I looked up at him for some response just as he batted my phone out of my hand onto the floor, pulling at the dogs again.

That was it.

I took a big stride forward, stepping over Red, and gave the bloke a big two-handed shove that sent him flying, roaring as loudly as I could, 'I said, pack it in!'

'Bobby!' Marie called out, and the dogs began to bark while running back to her and safety.

The Turkish guy scrambled to his feet, his fists clenching, but before he could find his balance, I pushed him again in the direction of the exit and went with him, grabbing his T-shirt in a tight ball under his neck with one hand as I caught his other arm trying to swing a punch. With several decades of rugby experience, I half lifted, half threw him back out of the entrance to the car park, then stood there panting, adrenaline going haywire through my body.

Welcome to Istanbul. It was the end of March, and we had arrived into a Turkey waking up to spring, after a slightly longer and more winding road than we'd originally planned.

We'd bumped our way into Albania seven weeks before and were quickly on roads that were more like tracks, with boulders, scrub and wild sage and thyme. We'd expected to be there for five days, but there was just so much to see, we stayed for twenty instead, driving through high mountains dusted with snow, snorkelling in water so blue it was like polished glass, riding horses through thickets of wind-roughened laurel and myrtle. We drove over blue misted hills that rolled in front of us like the swell of the sea. I even went spearfishing and managed to bag a moray eel. They aren't a nice thing to look at and it turns out they die *really* hard. This one was still wriggling after it had been gutted, cleaned and put on the barbecue. I took an apprehensive couple of bites and gave up, but Marie held her half in both hands and saw it off in seconds, reaching for my half too. Not one for me.

For Marie's twenty-ninth birthday, we went horse-trekking up steep mountain tracks – my way of thanking the mountains for bringing her to me. (This time was far less hazardous for my testicles.) It was perfect terrain for the truck, as we parked up alongside utterly deserted valleys, beaches and rivers. A large chunk of the time was spent with us bumping around the front of the truck like pinballs, music whacked up to eleven (Bob Dylan for me, some awful French music for her), and Marie and I singing along at the top of our lungs, while Red silently judged us. The rough roads took their toll on the truck, though, and we were forced into some more emergency repairs. Yet again, as Marie got stuck in, I was so grateful to be sharing this journey with someone who never felt sorry for herself and just got on with it.

As we crossed the border into Greece, I prayed the border guard wouldn't clock that I had exceeded my ninety-day maximum stay in the Schengen Zone – cheers, Brexit – as I saw him start to flick through the couple of dozen stamps we had collected up until now. Thankfully he soon gave up,

Truck It!

stamped my passport and threw it back out of the window at me.

We made our way lazily south, with no real plan, knowing only that we were meeting my dad and his partner Karen on the island of Kefalonia in March. One morning, we woke up to a drizzly spring day, went to do laundry at the nearest town and ended up in Corfu.

'We can literally go anywhere,' I giggled to Marie, who looked at me slightly confused. But I was dead serious. 'Let's do it! We can just play ferry roulette. Turn up to the port, book a ferry and see where we end up.'

By now, Marie had got used to the obscenely regular 'I've had an idea' moments. She'd also got used to telling me no. This time, however, two hours later, we were disembarking at Corfu's port.

But our fairy-tale, out-of-season exploration of deserted Greek islands was cut short when I noticed oil leaking from the prop shaft underneath the truck.

'She'll be alright. When it stops leaking, then we know we have a problem,' I declared, having spent years dispensing unwanted oil on friends' and family members' driveways from old Land Rovers.

Houston, we have a problem, I declared by text to my dad only twenty-four hours later when I went in for a closer inspection, sending him a video of the prop shaft, wobbling around. It was clear a bearing was collapsing.

A quick google, ferry journey, then a slow, nail-biting drive later, and we arrived at a rather run-down-looking MAN garage on the mainland, ready to have our pants pulled down and every last penny handed over.

Luckily, Nico and his lads at MAN Services in Patras not only solved our problem, but gave us a full tune-up for the next leg of the adventure. At the end of the three days, we handed over about half of what I was expecting to pay, in cash, before being gifted a huge bottle of homemade olive oil. The days that followed became a blur of beaches and saltwater, seafood and salad. We saw dolphins from the truck window, lay in bed on stunning beaches and spent hours exploring ancient partially buried cities from times gone by. We even found time to do a bit of skiing in Kalavryta.

In Kefalonia, we met my dad and Karen and took them on a surprise horse trek around the island to thank him for all the help on the truck build, while secretly stitching him up for the laugh.

'Have you ever been on a horse, Dad?' I said, knowing his answer.

'Yeah, I have actually. It was about thirty years ago, metal, and went round and around to music.'

He wasn't exaggerating. and about an hour later he tried to get on 'Megatron' backwards. It was amazing to see my dad again and show him the truck in action after we'd spent all that time together fitting it out.

I caught him one afternoon, opening a couple of the outside lockers he'd fitted himself, saying to a distinctly disinterested-looking Karen: 'Look at this, two-millimetre tolerance, perfect. I had to put some packers under there to level it so it closes perfectly along that edge, see?'

It was clear my dad was just as proud as I was to have been able to build a machine to take us to the far side of the world.

Truck It!

'Right, come on, little boy,' he said teasingly on the final day, after donning a pair of overalls he had brought with him. 'It's time for the old man to teach you some lessons. Get under here, let me show you how to adjust the brakes so you don't drive off a cliff in Pakistan.'

All too soon, it was time to hug my dad goodbye and set off back north.

We sped through North Macedonia, stopping only to hike the highest mountain, narrowly avoiding an avalanche, before being gifted an eye-wateringly expensive bottle of red wine by a nice gentleman who I was delicately told was the head of the local Mafia as he pulled away in his blacked-out BMW. As we were leaving, the waiter gave us a pen and invited us to write on the wall. Marie climbed on my shoulders and wrote: 'Life is beautiful, don't ever forget'. We drove about 200 miles east until, in a personally significant moment, we reached the ski town of Bansko at the foot of the Pirin mountains, which marked the furthest east I had ever been in my life.

It turned out that people in Bulgaria *really* like to drink.

On the first night, Marie got so blind drunk living her best life, eating too much cheese and drinking too much wine, that I had to put her to bed shortly after 10 p.m. An hour later I stood on the stage of the 'Amigo Pub' with the band, singing 'Sweet Caroline' to a packed club. Marie, to this day, still doesn't believe it happened.

Twenty-four hours later, almost to the minute, it was my turn to be put to bed – Marie helping me back to the truck in a nearby car park where we woke in the morning to a big stain all down its side, which we soon worked out was my vomit. Marie, rather than having gone to find a band to sing with, went and found a pizzeria and got stuck into a pizza, followed by a takeaway crêpe on the way back to a drunkenly passed-out Bobby.

Marie continued to get stuck in to absolutely everything we did, ate as much as me, drank as much as me, before out-dancing me on every dance floor we came across. No matter how empty the bar was or how sober we were, she would grab my hand and drag me, dancing her way onto the middle of the floor, before throwing it down with the execution of a professional dancer while I awkwardly two-stepped in front of her, laughing in awe.

However, we both decided that morning that we'd better not spend any more time in Bulgaria, if only for our livers' sakes, and made a quick departure towards Turkey.

Five hundred kilometres later, and we were sitting in a cafe, planning ahead. It was a smoky quiet place on the outskirts of the most intense city we had yet visited: Istanbul. Entering had been a complete assault on the senses as we fought our way through traffic, busier than anything we were used to. The noise, the smells, the sounds – everything was overwhelming, and we were fortunate to have found out about a small car park turned campervan spot just off the main highway through the city. We locked up and walked down to find an internet cafe.

We really had to work out some of the fundamentals of the next leg of our trip. Europe had been one thing, but much like travellers for thousands of years, by passing through Istanbul, we were about to symbolically enter Asia. And we needed to plot our route through to south-east Asia, where we'd eventually be shipping the truck to Australia. As we both plotted various routes on Google Maps, we compared notes.

'I think it's got to be Georgia, then Russia or Iran,' Marie said.

'No way, not Iran,' I said hurriedly. I had read about an overlander couple from New Zealand who had been detained for four months for no reason while crossing Iran. 'I know we shouldn't believe everything we read, but honestly with it all kicking off there I don't think it's right, plus we'd have to have a government escort at all times.'

'Do you not think Azerbaijan will open their borders? It's been a few years since Covid,' said Marie, which I laughed at, having just read about it on a forum.

'They've said they will open them three times, only to delay it each time. They did the same thing a few weeks ago. The theory is that the prime minister's wife is a major shareholder of Azerbaijan's biggest airline, which is profiting ludicrously, as the only way to get into the country is to fly in! Plus the quote to put the truck on a truck and take it over the border is extortionate. I'm not paying £7,000.'

'Okay, so it's Russia then,' said Marie.

'Guess so.'

'Okay, so with that sorted, what about after Tajikistan?' I enquired.

We both took a moment to let the question sink in while taking a chunk out of a Turkish delight and a swig of some awful Turkish tea.

'I'm still not sure about Afghanistan,' Marie said sheepishly.

'Yeah, but look, there hasn't been any war there for a while, and look at what other warnings we've had, and then had an incredible time. Romania – "don't go there, you'll get robbed, beat up, dogs stolen, truck parts nicked". It was the same for Albania,' I exclaimed, 'and they are our two favourite countries so far.'

Marie avoided eye contact and swilled the last of her tea full of grit.

'Look, it will cost thousands to cross around through China, which is somewhere I want to avoid as well, and we'd miss out on the Pamir Highway. Come on, let's at least look into it.'

Nervous but willing as ever, Marie nodded. 'Sure.'

'Okay, great! So, you're looking forward to being my wife then?'

That got Marie's attention.

'WHAT?' she squealed.

'It says here it looks like it might be possible from the Shir Khan Bandar border, where they issue visa-on-arrivals. They don't acknowledge any of their foreign embassies since the Taliban re-established themselves . . .' We both paused. 'But it looks like single women can't cross unaccompanied. They have to be chaperoned by a family member or husband. And I suspect your dad doesn't want to join us through Afghanistan.' We both laughed, slightly nervously to not jinx ourselves.

'Okay, yeah, fine, I guess,' said Marie slowly.

'Wait, I haven't asked for your hand in marriage yet; I'd better ring your dad. Come on, let's go for a nosey around the Grand Bazaar . . .'

We shut the laptops and headed off into the chaos and

touts with the dogs weaving their way through the foot traffic behind us, stopping every now and then to pee on the stall of a market seller, peddling counterfeited North Face clothes, who would chase after them both with a broom, much to their surprise and the amusement of onlookers.

'Four hundred pounds,' the big Turkish guy said, tapping the glass of the fake Rolex he was holding in my face. 'Very good price, my friend, very good.'

'A hundred. Honestly, mate, take it or leave it,' I said, laughing at his sales pitch.

'For you, special price,' he said, which set me off again. 'Two hundred. The best genuine fake in the whole of Turkey,' he proudly announced, and I laughed.

'My mum bought one of these a few years ago. The strap turned white after three days staining her skin, before the glass fell out and it stopped working two days later.'

'She did not buy from me then,' he declared.

I laughed and started to walk out: 'Alright, thanks, mate, but it's too much.'

We hadn't got five metres up the little alleyway in the vast labyrinth of the Grand Bazaar Market before hearing: 'My friend, come, just for you one hundred, but don't tell anybody. And leave the dogs outside, my friend is very scared.'

We smiled and walked back in, handed over the cash and proudly walked out with a shiny new genuine fake Rolex. And, to be fair, this particular one is still ticking away.

'I'll meet you at the bottom of the spice bazaar,' I told Marie afterwards. 'I said I'd call my mum about now. I won't be too long.'

Marie nodded, whistled for Rubia to follow and disappeared

off into the crowd with her personal bodyguard, who cleared a path like Moses parting the sea as locals jumped out of the way of what looked like a white wolf approaching. Marie strode confidently down the centre of the street.

I had spotted a rustic shop selling all sorts of hand-made, rusty, bent and badly engraved but beautiful jewellery and I thought it was the style perfectly suited for my wild and untameable nomadic French girlfriend.

I walked in hesitantly as a woman with a face covered in tattoos stood to greet me.

A few minutes later, I pointed: 'That one.' It was perfect: tarnished silver, not quite perfectly round, but engraved in a flowery pattern.

'How much?' I held my hand up and rubbed my finger and thumb together as the international sign.

She typed out sixteen on a calculator in front of her. Sixteen euros – was that right? I didn't want to give her a second chance, so handed over the cash, collected the ring and slipped it in a cute little ring bag and found Red sat waiting patiently outside.

'Is she okay?' asked Marie when we met up.

'Yeah, all good, just warned me not to get a fake Rolex,' I lied.

We both laughed, paid for the multiple bags Marie had been busy filling with all sorts of colourful-looking spices, and set off back to the truck. We had just arrived back and I was unlocking the back when the skinny Turkish guy had suddenly grabbed the dogs' leads.

'Go on! Piss off!' I shouted after successfully freeing them and chucking him out of the car park. Eventually the dog

Truck It!

violator got the message that he had picked on the wrong couple and scurried away before I turned to the two security guards who, upon hearing the commotion, had taken precisely half a step out of their cabin, both still holding their takeaway kebabs in a polystyrene box.

'Lads, what the hell?' I shrugged loudly in their direction.

Knowing it was a waste of time to do absolutely anything other than pull the gate shut to the makeshift campervan park-up, I walked back to the truck to make a fuss of the dogs, who were still looking a little shocked.

'What the hell was that about?' said Marie, as I got attacked with concerned licks from both dogs.

'Absolutely no idea. Let's just be a bit more careful with the kids while we're here and keep the truck properly locked up. He's the type of guy to come back and set fire to the truck just because he can.'

That night, we all slept with one eye open.

The second and final day in Istanbul, we went to invest in some new climbing boots, making sure these were the genuinely article, before popping to get some missing spear-fishing kit (now I was turning professional, having begun catching specimens larger than goldfish). The shop owner couldn't stop recommending 'His' island.

'It's paradise. You must go,' he insisted after we told him of our travels.

'I guess we are going to paradise island then,' we giggled together, walking back into the city for the final night in search of some good kebab to gorge on.

After a rooftop meal of Turkish delight, we had a tray of baklava, which we consumed sat on the quay, looking over at the far side of the river marking the start of the Asian continent.

The past six months travelling south and east through Europe had been incredible, from warm blue seas to high white mountains and everything in between. But we both knew that we were properly changing gears now. We headed back through the dark alleys of Istanbul towards the truck and dogs who we had left on guard inside.

We criss-crossed through dark alleyways, full of stray dogs and plastic packaging from the fake gear being sold by the tonne to European tourists making their yearly pilgrimage to the counterfeit Mecca of the world.

Here, I thought, *it's dark enough to not draw too much attention*, stopping beside a small mosque and the bins.

Without grabbing Marie's attention, I dropped to one knee, pulled out the ring I had been carrying nervously all night, and called out her name as she had walked ahead a few paces.

'Marie . . .'

'Oh, how romantic,' she giggled.

'Will you be my Afghan wife?'

'Oh yes, yes!'

She grabbed my face with both hands and gave me a big, sarcastic cartoon kiss on the lips.

I rose and slowly slid the ring on the finger she was pointing in my direction.

We laughed and continued to walk, hand in hand towards the truck.

'Oh bugger,' I let out quietly, looking in the direction of a shopkeeper who had been lurking in the shadows of his shop a few metres away.

Truck It!

He was now wearing the biggest smile, having just seen what he thought was a life-changing moment in our lives. As we approached, he began vigorously clapping and shouted, 'Congratulations!'

We both laughed so hard we couldn't walk straight.

12

Ups and Downs

'*Merde, putain.* Bobby, look!'

Marie had a habit of reverting to 50 per cent French swearwords in stressful moments.

I turned around and heard a loud roaring as a huge hot-air balloon came floating past us only a few metres away. It was almost close enough to touch, lit up bright by its burner, only narrowly missing us as it began to drop down past the cliff we were parked on. In the valley below, it joined with a hundred other hot-air balloons falling and rising in the dark purple sky above the jagged plateau that stretched in front of us.

We sat with a gentle wind at our backs, our feet dangling over the edge of the truck's roof, watching the gas burners firing into the lightening sky. It was just before 6 a.m. and

Truck It!

we were in Cappadocia, a district in Anatolia in Turkey. Marie, my mum and her partner Stephen and I had been watching as balloons in the distance flickered like Christmas decorations then risen into the sky. I'd managed to convince them that the best views were from this cliff on a ridge at the side of the valley, rather than stood shoulder to shoulder in a basket with fifty tourists, or huddled like penguins below. But we had no idea that the deserted cliff face we'd park up at was so close to where some took off. As we'd sat, more than a dozen came within touching distance of us.

'Oh, Bobby. It's amazing,' said my mum, her glasses hanging off the edge of her nose as she outstretched her arms, squinting to take a picture.

'That was one of the most beautiful things I've ever seen,' said Stephen, his voice a little choked up. 'Thank you for inviting us here.'

My mum and Stephen had been so supportive during the worst period of my life and I was so grateful to share this with them. I struggled to keep control of my own wobbly lower lip.

Marie and I had arrived two days earlier, having spent the past month after leaving Istanbul bouncing down the west coast of Turkey. In a ferry terminal in Izmir, a bustling port town on the Aegean, a guy smoking an enormous cigar and leaning back on his chair promised that he would 'make' the truck fit on his ferry with the slurred confidence of a man who'd enjoyed some beers with lunch. We had decided to take some time hopping between the North Aegean islands just off the west coast of Turkey but are actually part of

Greece. At first, we were told the ferry was full, only to have him call from the back office.

'How big? How heavy?'

'Seven metres, ten tonne,' I responded.

'No problem. Two hours, don't be late.'

I waved thanks, then sheepishly paid the ticket vendor who was clearly pissed off at being overruled. I walked out to Marie and explained what had just happened.

'So how big is this ferry?'

'No idea. A car ferry, I presume. It sounds like we only just fit on. It must be busy.'

One hour and fifty-five minutes later, having officially stamped out of Turkey into 'no-man's water', and now in a slight tizz given how last-minute we were running because of another shit show of a border, we drove up to a guy waving in our direction, pointing to a gap at the quay between two big ships.

'Oh my god, no way,' said Marie.

I was stumped. Physically speechless.

'Do you want me to guide you in?' Marie asked, realizing how tight a space we had to fit in.

I dithered to say something. I was trying to decide whether we should cancel the crossing there and then.

Marie hopped out, passing me a walkie-talkie as I shouted out of the window: 'Marie, I just don't think we actually fit. Like it doesn't look long enough . . .'

The 'ship' docked in front of us with its ramp down in our direction was about the size of a ferry normally seen on Lake Windermere. It was certainly not a proper ferry. More of a metal dinghy. There were two small cars already on the deck

Truck It!

and three people all stood in shock as I started to edge my way forward under the direction of Marie and the drunken cigar-smoker we had seen a few hours earlier.

'Marie, keep an eye on the waterline,' I shouted helplessly into the radio as it felt like the tin can wouldn't take our weight.

We shuffled forward, back, back off, back on, forwards, until the captain gave up and ordered a couple of lads to bring straps and the buoys normally used on the outside of the boat and wedged them against the cab of the truck to stop it bashing the guard rail.

Then they set about strapping the truck down to the boat – not with ratchets, but with old salt-damaged rope. One guy chose the fuel tank on one side to tie us down to. The other chose the retracted steps, which he clearly didn't realize would simply open if any force was applied.

I was too distracted to say anything though, as I was watching the captain pull the ramp up under the back of the truck.

'It doesn't shut,' I informed him, helpfully.

'No problem,' he mumbled around the cigar hanging out of the side of his mouth.

The ramp pulled up just above the waterline where he stopped it, closed the switch cover and walked to the front of the boat.

Marie caught my eye. We both shook our heads.

'Let's open the truck cab windows,' I whispered, 'so if we do sink, at least the dogs can get out.' Marie scrambled in to give the unwilling seadogs an escape route.

At one point during the crossing, the captain suddenly appeared at our side.

'Okay?' he shouted over the noise of the engine, wind and sea.

'Hope so,' Marie shrugged back.

El Capitano made a prayer sign across his chest before running back to the wheel he should probably have been holding on to, especially given the state of the waves.

For a half-hour that felt like days, we prayed, pointed and winced as the truck swayed violently, its wheels lashed by sea water that washed up the partially closed ramp. The dogs stared helplessly out at us.

I don't think I blinked for the whole crossing. My knuckles were white with tension when we finally entered the port on the island of Chios. That night, we answered every situation with a mumbled 'no problem' as we drank freezing cold local beer until we finally calmed down.

For the next couple of weeks, we wild-camped on white sandy beaches under permanently blue skies. We swam and snorkelled. We ate at local restaurants or caught fish and barbecued it on the beach, eating it with our hands minutes after we'd pulled it from the water. We swam and slept and at night lay and looked up at the stars. When we could fit, we squeezed onto ferries, sometimes being told only at the last minute we'd have to get off at the next port. On one island, we were told about an old guy who'd turned an abandoned house from a deserted mountain village into a restaurant whose menu simply read: 'Meat or no meat. Wine or Beer'.

When we arrived, there was a guy playing traditional music on a guitar. Before any drinks were served, the other diners got stuck straight into the night's festivities, climbed onto their tables, threw napkins and smashed plates. Marie and I sat gawping from a quiet corner as the waiter/owner mounted another chair, cigarette hanging out of the side of his mouth, to throw another stack of napkins at the group of Greek locals doing a clearly well-practised dance in a circle.

'Where are you going?' I said to Marie as she got up.

But it was too late, and she skipped towards the circle of dancers, who welcomed her in, laughing. I marvelled again at her ability to jump into any situation.

Soon, however, it was finally time to head back to the mainland, and one only mildly less terrifying ferry crossing later, we were back on dry land. We would need to travel more than a thousand miles east to the Turkish/Georgian border, but before that we had our very special rendezvous with my mum and Stephen.

After we'd seen the balloons, we spent a couple of days exploring the astonishing valleys in the area, ones that looked like the surface of another planet. But then it was time to go. As we were fuelling up before heading east, we bumped into a couple driving an old and very beaten-up beige SUV with all sorts hanging off it. Out came a shaggy-haired bloke who proceeded to say 'nice truck' with a strong Geordie accent. Marie came over and Tyler's girlfriend, Poppy, came out and we all got talking. They had originally taken a year off to backpack in south-east Asia, but had gotten bored of the tourist trail and decided to buy a vehicle and drive to eastern Russia. For the first time, I felt what many others must have thought when I explained where we planned on driving. I smiled and politely wished them the best of luck before getting back in and raising my eyebrows at Marie.

'Tenner says they don't make it.'

We hadn't made it very far ourselves through the west of central Turkey when I tried to change gear as we reached the crest of a hill and just couldn't. The gearstick just flopped around. I coasted to the side of the road and put the hazards on.

'What's going on?' Marie looked over at me, worried.

'Honestly no idea, but whatever it is, it's not good.'

We were on the outskirts of a nondescript town, having just bounced our way over a rough track through deep channels cut by water.

'Hold on, I think I've got it,' I said. Using two hands, I was able to force the gearstick in place, then move it into gear, but when I let go it collapsed forward.

'I think the technical term is knackered,' I said.

We crawled for a couple of miles in first gear until we found somewhere safer to pull in, near what looked like a stable.

I called my dad and over the next half an hour we went through all the various things that might have gone wrong. Finally, he reminded me that a very heavy stone arch had fallen on the truck in Italy. I thanked him for that reminder, then lifted up the cab and crawled underneath to poke around.

'There's a snapped bracket!' I shouted in joy.

'Is that good?' said Marie.

'Well, no. But I can fix it at least.' I looked over at the building. 'Maybe they have a welder they would be willing to lend to a damsel in distress?' I said, with puppy-dog eyes.

Truck It!

She just laughed and headed off.

Five minutes later, three guys were setting up an electrical extension and a mini welder as I got back underneath with a grinder to clean up the bracket ready for welding.

'Do you need help? We can call a mechanic or welder?' said the owner of the horse ranch.

'Nah,' I assured them, 'it's all good. It only needs to last until we get a new part.' I pulled down the visor and set about welding. When I was finished, I asked how much we owed them and they just held their palms out.

'Please, no, this is our gift. Welcome to Turkey. You are our guest, and we are thankful we can help you.' We thanked them profusely and set off. The gearstick seemed to be back to normal for now.

For two and a half long, featureless days we moved east through dry barren scrubland in various shades of beige and brown. At one point we stopped at a reservoir to cool the dogs down and saw the spear of a mosque poking out, so went to explore. We swam over to it and walked on the top of walls from the houses in the valley they'd flooded to make the reservoir while the dogs swam between the 'rooms' half a metre below us. Later we read that it was called Halfeti, and had been flooded in 1999 to make the Birecik Dam.

As we got back to the truck, Marie called back to me: 'Bobby, there's someone snooping around.'

I caught up and crossed the empty highway to find a big bullish-looking guy sizing up the truck. He was dressed in scruffy clothes and had an impatient look on his dirty face. He said a word in Turkish.

'Ummm . . .' I replied.

Then he pointed to the grinder he was holding. 'Power,' he said. 'Come.'

He grabbed my arm under my armpit and marched me round the corner where a big truck was abandoned on the side of the road with its wheel hanging off at a forty-five-degree angle, its driver relaxing in the shade.

'All good,' I called to Marie. 'He's a mechanic. There's a broken down truck. I'm going to try to give them a hand.'

'Here.' I passed him my electric battery grinder, which was received with a big grin, and got stuck in with him.

We wrestled the old tyre off, stripped the hub to reveal the collapsed wheel bearing, which set the mechanic off swearing – the universal first step of any repair job in any language.

What was more surprising was the way that he treated Marie.

'Three coffee,' he said without looking up at her and in a tone of voice that took us both back. It was the first time we'd encountered something people had warned us about for this next stage of our trip. Marie brought the coffees to me and said, 'I'm not giving it to them. Wankers.' And walked off.

As we were sat in the shade, waiting, two young lads came over who had been hitchhiking in the truck when it had broken down. They were shy, and though they were far too young to smoke, cadged a fag off the driver, who spent the whole time smoking in the shade of a tree.

'Climbing?' I said to them, miming, as they smiled shyly back. I went and got a climbing rope from the back of the truck and tossed it over the edge of the bridge we were

Truck It!

parked next to, then tied it off. It was about a twenty-metre drop down to a valley below. I then went and got Marie's climbing harnesses and one of mine. I beckoned to one of them. 'Come,' I said. They were both laughing and shaking their heads but clearly really excited.

Using broken English and mime, I showed them how to belay, while tugging at the second line that I controlled to demonstrate that they weren't at any risk of falling. Then the first kid climbed into the harness and climbed over the edge of the bridge. Slowly, I encouraged him, and showed him how to lean backwards over the edge. 'You've got this,' I said. He leaned back, laughing before he was fully over, shrieking with a mixture of joy and fear. His mate could hardly film him, he was laughing so hard. Finally he got to the bottom and came scrambling up the bank, breathless, clearly telling his mate how much fun it was. Then they swapped. As he leaned back over the edge, a pickup full of workers slowed down to see what was going on, and all jumped out laughing and clapping as they watched this young lad rappel himself down. Finally, the truck was fixed and it was time for them to leave. The two boys shook my hand, placing the other hand over their heart as they thanked me.

'You come tea,' the mechanic said, holding a business card with the address of a garage on it. 'Come,' he insisted.

'Okay,' I laughed, looking at Marie for approval. 'Tomorrow.'

He shook my hand with a grip strong enough to break a finger and in a puff of black smoke was gone.

I looked up the address and it was in a town right next to the border with Georgia. 'It is on the way,' I said.

'Aaaaaaaaaah!' roared the mechanic standing on top of the

truck when he saw us the next morning. The other mechanics stopped, then wiped their hands and came over. He shouted at a younger lad, handed over cash and pointed him out of the garage.

No one spoke English and we didn't have a Turkish word to share between us, but with hand gestures and Google Translate, we both laughed at what we ended up doing yesterday.

'Can you have a look at something for me?' I typed into the translator, at which the guy scowled and waved, 'come on'.

I showed him pictures of the bad weld and broken part, which sent him into a tizz. He waved all the mechanics to move some parts out of the way before one of the lads started to grab a tool to lift our cab while others grabbed some ladders and started bringing over a tray of tools.

Twenty minutes later, four mechanics and a welder from next door had the bracket off, welded back properly, sprayed up, replaced and cab back down, just as the young lad returned carrying two trays of cups of tea and two carrier bags full of polystyrene takeaway bags, looking extremely flustered.

'Come, eat,' the guy said, slapping me hard enough on my back to knock out any false teeth I might have had.

We all sat in a little timber shack in the back of the garage and tucked into kebab, tea and bread at what must have been 10 a.m. My kind of guys.

As someone started tidying up, he handed me his phone that displayed a translated message: 'Please join me and my family tonight. You are our guests. We want to take you to our favourite restaurant.'

Truck It!

Shocked and taken aback, I turned to Marie and in unison we nodded and agreed: 'Okay, sure!'

While the guys got back to work, we wandered around Hopa, which was full of thousands, literally *thousands*, of heavy-set truck drivers, waiting to cross into Georgia. 'But these guys are all driving Azerbaijan, Kazakhstan and Uzbek trucks,' I said into the translation app, and passed it over to the driver we were walking round with.

'Yes. Azerbaijan border shut and they do not let in. Everyone waits here in a queue and then crosses into Georgia in a line and heads to the border. Turkey is much better for the drivers, so everyone waits here and sets off when they are told.'

I couldn't believe it. I knew the borders were disorganized but to see a whole town completely rammed full of drivers, a whole country away from where they were going, was a sight to behold. There were trucks with huge trailers bursting with goods on every piece of available tarmac. Cars weaved around them as if it were completely normal.

'So much for crossing today,' Marie joked as we turned up at the restaurant a few hours later.

The mechanics had scrubbed up as best mechanics are able to do, with oil under their fingernails and wild, dust-filled hair.

'My wife, my friend's wife,' said the big guy as we all sat down to what was to be a fantastic evening of platters of meat and bread, which we dipped into garlicky yoghurt and hummus, enjoying the delicious local booze and lots of laughter as we all told stories through our translation app. Throughout the whole evening, each one of us held a fork in one hand, the other hand typing away vigorously on a phone trying to keep up with the conversation.

'Okay, how much do we owe you?' I said at the end of the meal. 'The repair, tea, food and tonight.'

The guy leaned back in his chair waving both hands in front of his chest.

His friend and business partner typed away next to him and passed me a message that read: 'You are our guests, please, it is our pleasure to host you. Remember us when you drive around the world. We wish you all the best of luck.'

Our time in this country had begun with me shouting at the top of my lungs, but ended with me utterly grateful for the kindness of strangers. However, as we reached mid-May and the promise of summer was louder in the air with every day that passed, it was time to enter the complete unknown that was Georgia.

13

Snow Problem

'Bobby! Run!'

I looked up to see the avalanche bearing straight down the mountain towards us. I scrambled to my feet, slipping as I took a handful of Marie's jacket and dragged her behind the truck.

'Everyone, behind the truck, now!'

I watched as Tyler grabbed the spare wheel and jack. 'Leave it. Get here, now!'

As the first clods of snow began to hit the side of the truck, Tyler arrived, sliding into us. The truck wobbled and snow began to pile over and under it, all around us, and I prayed to a god I didn't believe in that the pressure from the snow didn't push us all off into the abyss.

Welcome to Georgia.

Bobby Bolton

At first, it had been a relief to leave the arid, dry environment of Turkey. It had rained the first day we arrived, but then it didn't stop for two weeks. It was like Wigan, but without the pies. We drove past villages where pigs, cows, goats and chickens roamed free. Kids played in the field and fishermen cast their rods into the lazy river next to lush green fields. But it soon became clear that, as well as the good weather, we had also left the friendliness of Turkey behind.

In Turkey, pretty much every time we stopped, someone would come and say hello and ask us what we were doing. The first time we stopped just over the border in Georgia, I called out 'hello' to someone walking down the street, only for them to cross to the other side to avoid me. As the days passed and we continued to be met with the same mixture of suspicion, disinterest and sometimes outright hostility, I began to wonder what the problem was.

A backpacker we met called Joo Won, who was from Korea, explained to us that Russia had invaded Georgia in 2008 and was still in control. 'They did it to stop Georgia joining the European Union,' he said, tucking into a massive bowl of dumplings. 'You can see anti-Russian graffiti everywhere.' I resolved to be a bit more understanding of their suspicion of strangers from now on.

If the people were a little standoffish, however, the scenery, at least, was astonishing. As we drove through the Caucasus mountains, tiny clusters of villages like Mestia and Ushguli nestled in the rich green, with mountains looming dark behind them. We drove over winding mountain roads, down into valleys, past deep rivers surrounded by the green grass and trees, and then up into the blinding white of the snow

Truck It!

mountains. There were ancient stone buildings and drystone walls clinging to the sides of the valley, carved out by glaciers, and thousand-year-old stone watchtowers lined the ridges, standing guard. The villages were mazes of steep muddy paths, while the biggest dogs I have ever seen roamed to keep guard against the wolves in the mountain forests.

The only drama was when my boy Red was attacked by one of these giant mountain dogs, who locked his jaws around his neck and wouldn't let go. I was forced to kick 'Dogzilla' until he let go, then throw him over the edge of the path. Even as we ran away, the huge animal began to lumber back up the bank.

We agreed to meet up with Poppy and Tyler the Geordie a few days later, before they crossed into Russia. We compared notes on the hassles of getting into Russia and agreed to drive in convoy over a high mountain pass. They were behind us, when at one point they started waving and slowing down. I ran back up to them as they came to a stop and said they'd got a flat tyre. On one side of us was a mountainside of snow and ice, the other a steep drop. We weighed up the dangers and decided that the lack of traction with a flat on that surface, with a drop to the side, was just too risky. We'd change the tyre there. I was halfway between the truck and their jacked-up Mercedes SUV when the avalanche started.

For what felt like a lifetime but was only seconds, the truck kept rocking as the snow piled up as we hid behind it. Then the rumble stopped and silence once again took over as we held our breaths. We peeked around. It was finished. Poppy started to laugh in relief.

'Christ, that was lucky. Wouldn't have needed to be much

more force to have us over the cliff,' I said. We went and looked at their Mercedes, which was half-buried. Frantically we dug for a few minutes to uncover its front right tyre, which had been pushed off the jack by the avalanche, before resetting it and working to change the tyre as quickly as any Formula One team.

Poppy stood on guard looking up into the clouds for signs of any more snow, while Marie went to check on the dogs.

The truck ploughed a route through the fresh mound of snow for the Mercedes to follow, which in our haste had its front bumper and registration number plate ripped off. We didn't bother to stop to recover them.

Later that evening, we washed away the anxiety with a couple of pints of beer around a campfire.

'That's the last time we ever follow you up into the mountains,' laughed Tyler as he prodded the fire. They had received their travel paperwork, but we were yet to, so while we waited for our visa appointment, we explored more of the countryside. At roadside stalls they would slap freshly made dough against the inside of the hot ovens before it was peeled off and served straight to you. It is probably the best bread I've ever eaten. The only danger was that if one of you went to buy one to share, you'd already eaten half by the time you got back to the truck.

One afternoon, a few days before we were hoping to cross the border, we got a text from the visa centre.

Send picture of your white truck.

'Bobby, have you seen this? What do they mean "white truck"?'

'Oh, bloody hell,' I sighed, dropping tools and rolling out

Truck It!

from under the truck, where I was giving the vehicle a once-over and adding more plates of metal to patch up our long-suffering ride.

'I didn't think they would pick up on it. The insurance people at the border of Turkey questioned it but I just shrugged it off.' I sighed, ready to explain. 'Basically, the truck is still registered as a truck with a water bowser on the back. I painted it at the start of the conversion but ran out of time and effort before leaving the UK, so didn't bother updating the registration documents to a blue campervan.'

'You're kidding,' said Marie, who squatted down in the shade next to me. 'So, what are we going to do?'

I scoffed – it was a laugh of 'I don't know and can't be bothered'.

'Tell you what,' I said as I got back underneath the truck, 'can you text them back a photo of the truck now? It's got the right reg. Maybe it will suffice.'

'Bobby! They've replied!' Marie shouted over the noise of the grinder a short while later.

'What did they say?' I lifted my eye protection and turned to look at her through the chassis rails.

'"Send photo of the white truck from the application. Closing time 4 p.m." I don't think they speak much English,' said Marie sheepishly. 'It's just after two now and the office is about an hour and a half away.'

I laughed, sagging my head to the floor with my arms still holding the grinder and pieces of metal I was cutting to make fit.

'Alright, come on, let's pack up as quick as we can. Just throw all the tools in. I'm not paying for another visa application and waiting another two or three weeks. We don't have that long left on our visa in Georgia. This needs sorting pronto!'

'How?'

'We'll paint the truck.'

'Bobby, we've only got like an hour and a half.'

'We'd better be quick then, hadn't we? Come on.'

I grabbed a couple of bolts and zip ties and temporarily half-fitted a two-metre section of metal I hadn't yet finished cutting and drilling into place. As we drove down the dirt track in search of a builders' merchants, the rear habitation box was held on with the grand total of four substantially undersized bolts, just down one side.

'Are you sure?' Marie said, grabbing her seat as we bounced slowly through a river and re-joined the main road.

'If we don't get this approved, we are completely snookered. We'll have to go back to Turkey and work out a way of re-applying, or we'll have to fly home.' The impatience was making me drive faster than I should have been.

'There,' shouted Marie, fifteen minutes later down the valley.

We abandoned the truck outside a builders' merchants on the edge of the road, and ran in.

We grabbed a tub of white paint, a roller, and a couple of brushes.

'Hello, do you speak English?' I said.

'Yes, a small bit,' said the friendly but unenthusiastic shop owner.

'Do you mind if we pay for this later? We might need more. We have to repaint the truck,' I said, pointing to the

Truck It!

blue truck parked outside on the road, which got him to raise an eyebrow.

I explained the full circumstance, hoping it might get him on side. 'Show me,' he said as he walked out from behind his plywood desk.

I dropped the kit and walked outside, growing slightly more impatient as time ticked by.

'We have to paint the whole truck. It doesn't need to be a good job. I'll repaint it when we are out of Russia,' I said.

He didn't say anything and walked back into the shop. Marie and I looked at each other slightly confused. He appeared a couple of moments later holding a bottle of white spirit and an old rag.

He walked up to the door of the truck, applied a generous amount to the rag, and started rubbing.

My jaw dropped as the blue paint began to come away to reveal the factory original white paint.

'NO way! You genius,' I declared, patting him on the back.

'I'll go and grab some more,' said Marie as she followed the owner back inside the shop.

I set up a little extendable ladder I had stored on the truck, when Marie appeared with an armful of rags, white spirit and gloves.

'Let's get cracking,' I said, climbing the ladder and rubbing furiously.

'I think I might start on the back,' I said twenty minutes later.

But the shopkeeper waved a hand and said, 'Hold on. I don't know if you need to do that. A white truck is just the front. The back is like a trailer.'

'Good point,' I said, accepting his point of view nervously. 'But I don't want to take the risk. I'd rather do it all.'

'Give me five minutes,' he said, putting down his rag and disappearing off to make a call.

A few minutes later he returned. 'It's okay, just the front. My brother works for the government. I'm not too sure doing what, but he's important. He said is just front for colour.'

'Holy shit. Alright, let's go with that,' I said, raising my eyebrows as Marie turned to me, giving me an 'are you sure?' look.

'Let's focus on the front and get that neater,' I said as twenty past three approached.

'That'll do,' I announced as the guy and Marie stood back. I took a photo of a white fronted-truck with blue sides and pressed send.

'Alright, let's carry on just in case,' I said, still determined.

A few minutes later we got a text: **Thank you.**

'Does that mean we don't need to do the sides?' Marie called to me, up on the ladder.

'No idea, but I'm not taking more risk. Plus, we can't drive around with a multicoloured cab. Let's finish off the sides and call it there.'

At 3.50 p.m. I took two more tactical photos of just the cab, which was now white with the odd smear of blue, and pressed send. No response.

'Well, let's pray they got it and that will do,' I said as we stood paying for all the empty bottles of white spirit and rags, now strewn around the truck. We settled up, shook hands, thanked the guy profusely, and set off back to the mountain field to carry on with the metalwork under the chassis.

Truck It!

Your passport is ready for collection, read a text message that came through on what was a beautiful early May morning.

'Does that mean it's approved or rejected?' said Marie, a little confused.

I pondered the question for a few minutes. 'Shit, that sounds like a refusal. Surely it would say it's approved if it had been?' I said.

Marie tried to cheer me up. 'No, come on, it's approved. That's just a standard text.'

I was tired from working all weekend readying the truck for what I thought would be some of the worst driving roads in the world.

Three hours later, just before closing time, we were sitting in the visa centre waiting to be seen.

'Shhhhhhh,' said the fierce-looking Russian receptionist as she chatted loudly with her friend.

Having been called forward to collect my visa, I was talking to an Australian family who sat looking extremely nervous waiting to submit their own application to cross Russia in three days. They had the same plan as us.

'Shhhhh!' she said again. 'Or you will be kicked out.' We had been whispering bits of advice back and forth but promptly shut up.

'Mr Bolton?' said a deep Russian voice. I felt like I was in a James Bond movie. 'Visa approved. Start in two days. Three days to cross the country and get into Kazakhstan.'

I shrank into my chair, turned to Marie who was still sat waiting in the reception area, gave her a thumbs-up and mouthed, 'It's been approved.'

We both skipped out of there, ecstatic that we'd just

navigated a make-or-break moment, but very aware that our respective countries were on the other side of a war with the country we were about to enter. We agreed to keep our heads down, take the Instagram tag off the truck, not post on social media while we were there or do anything that might draw attention to us. There would be no sightseeing, just a straight shot 400 miles north and east through southwest Russia and up into Kazakhstan.

The night before crossing, as nerves were peaking, we decided to park up near the border, grab some food and discuss what the next few days looked like. I spotted a small track leading off through the bushes towards a wide, slow river. We splashed through a couple of puddles, past some piles of rubbish, to where the vegetation gave way to rocky shoreline.

'Mmmm, I'm not sure, let's head back to the main field,' I said, starting to make a three-point down the narrow muddy track. I went to drive forwards. 'Oh no. No. Not now . . .'

'What is it?' said Marie. We were stuck. In the dark I had reversed blindly up onto a bank of mud and become completely wedged, burying the transfer case, fuel tank and rear axle.

We tried all the tricks, reduced the tyre pressure and made the situation substantially worse as it dropped the truck's belly even deeper into the mud, which I then cocked up further by spinning the wheels with impatience and dug the truck in even further. For the first time, I felt like crying. I was so tired, hungry and pissed off. We'd spent the past day in Georgia hiking high into the snowy mountains, burning some energy in anticipation of three marathon

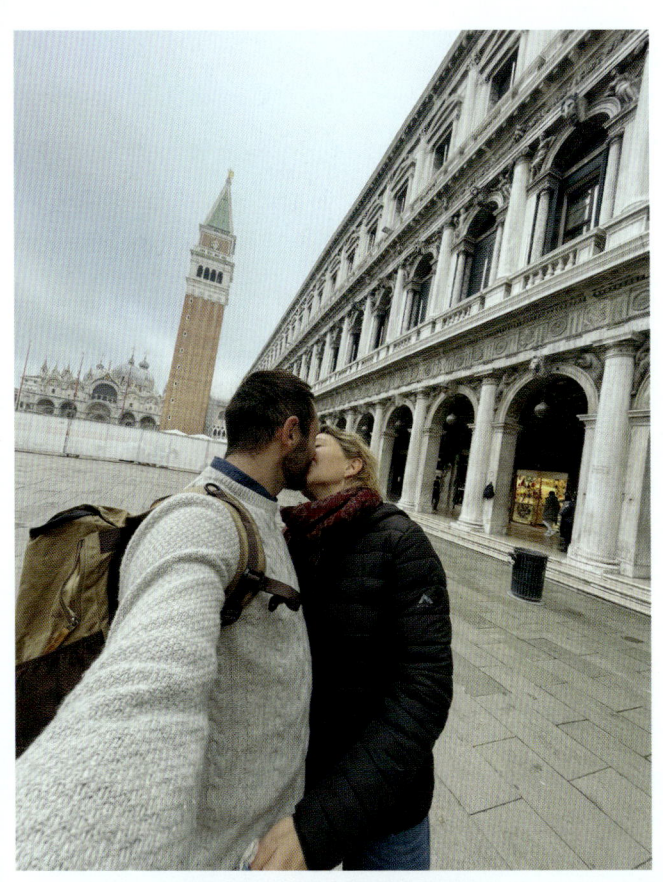

November 2023, Italy. Asking Marie to be my girlfriend in St Mark's Square, Venice. Fifty years on from when my grandparents visited for their honeymoon.

Red and Rubia getting to know each other better as our family of four set off on this crazy adventure.

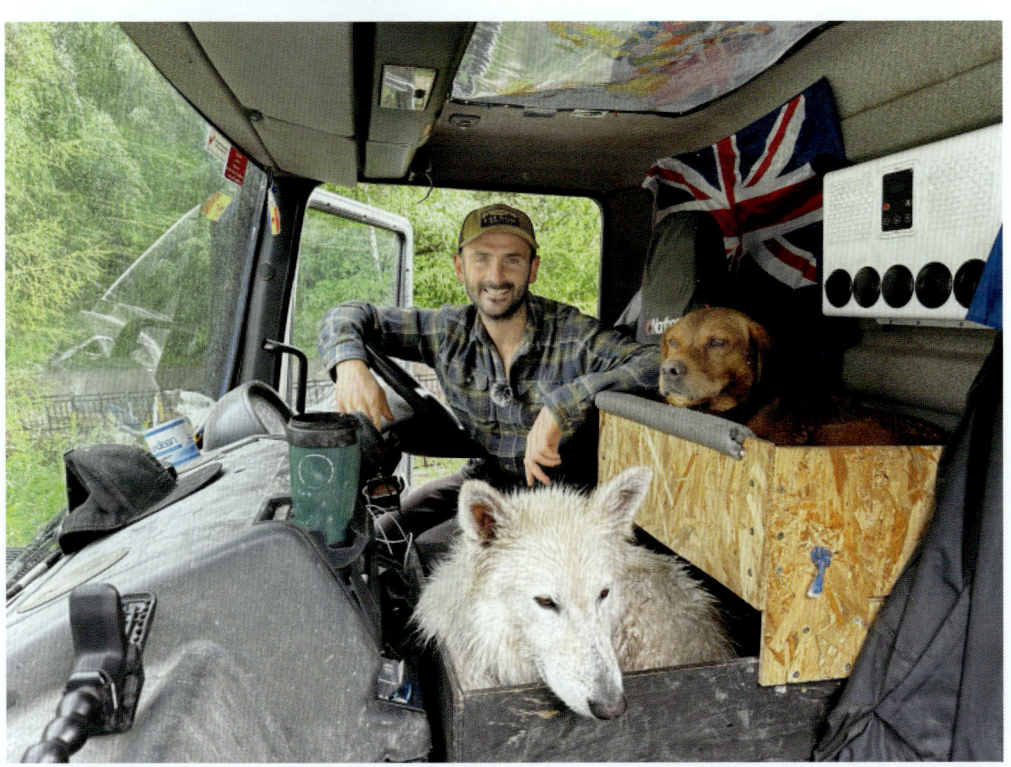

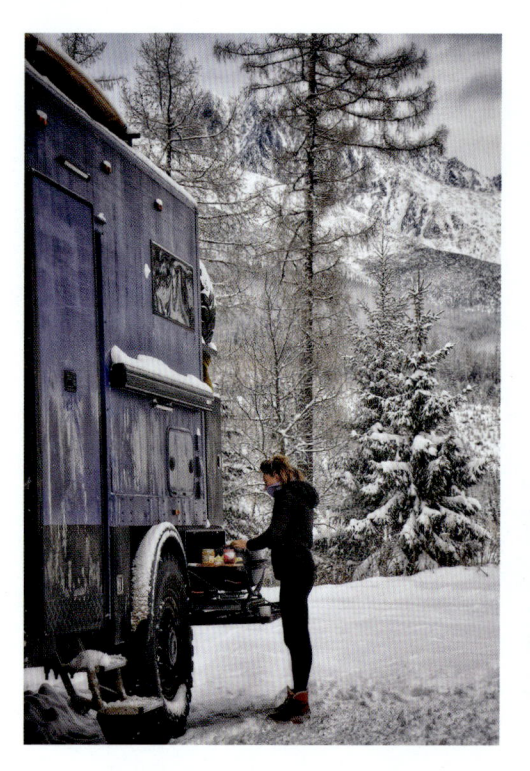

November 2023, Slovakia. Marie cooks toast for breakfast on the outside BBQ in the snow.

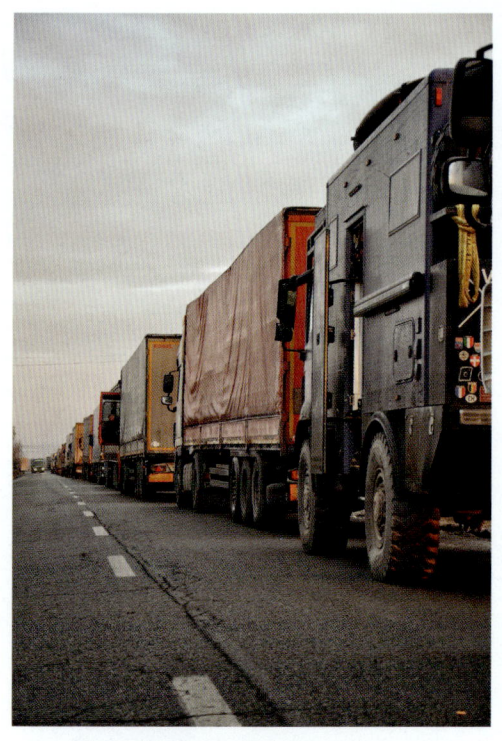

December 2023, Moldovan border. Practising our patience as we queue to leave the EU.

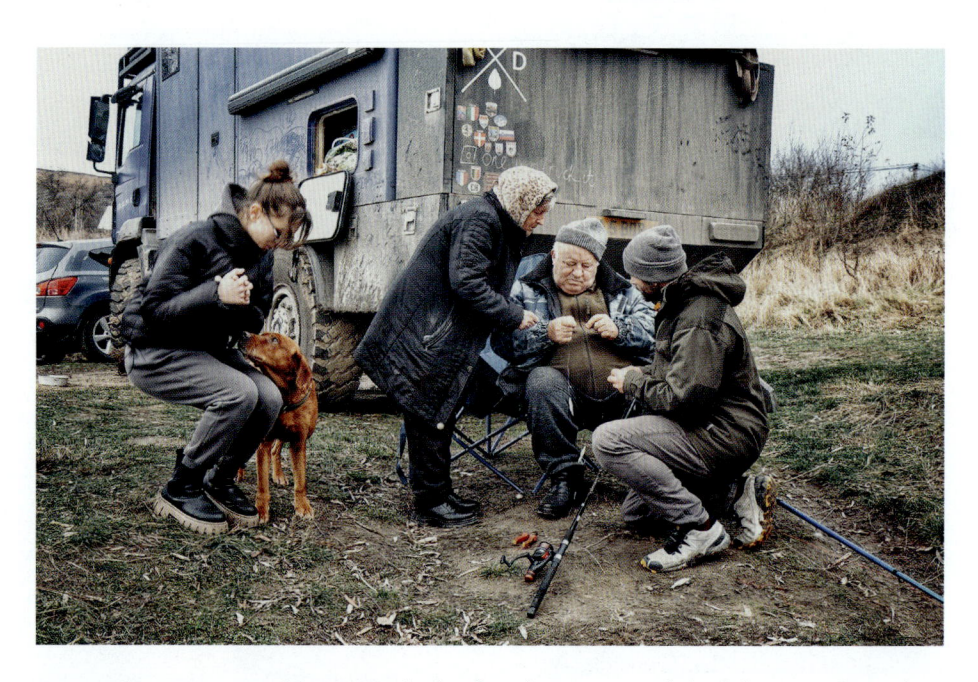

December 2023, Moldova. With the family we met while fishing with Sasha. This family spent an hour chatting with us, before disappearing and returning with local food, which we all enjoyed on a camping table outside the truck.

January 2024, Bosnia.
Ski-touring through the
mountains with the dogs
who LOVED it!

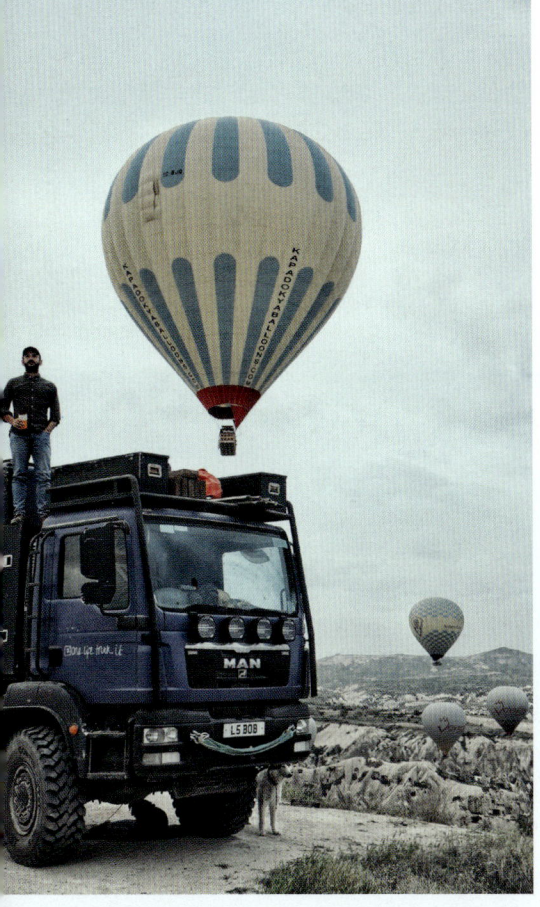

April 2024, Turkey.
Watching the balloons rise
over the moon-like landscape
at sunrise in Cappadocia.

June 2024, Georgia.
Stuck overnight in deep,
boggy ground as we prepared
to cross into Russia.

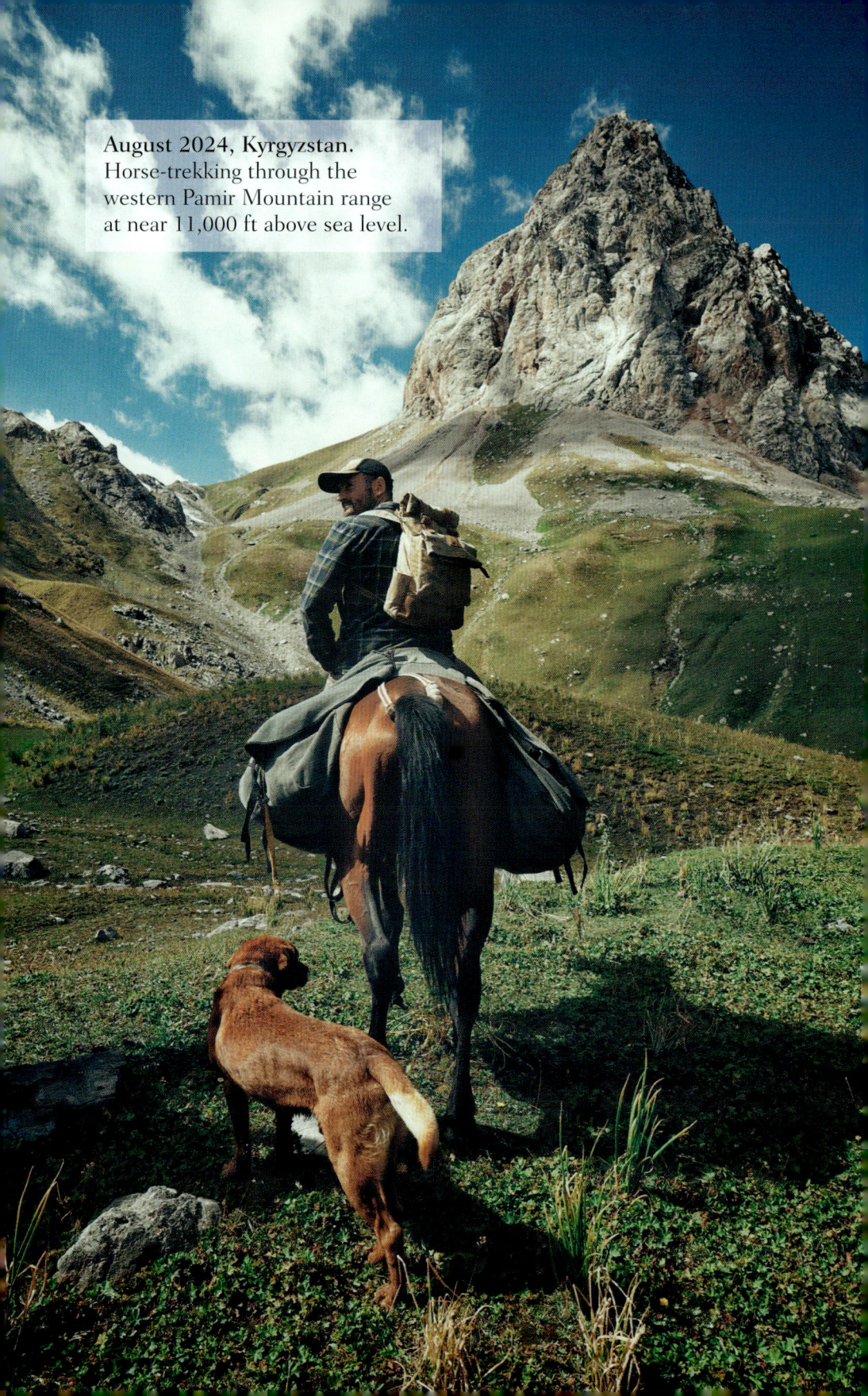

August 2024, Kyrgyzstan. Horse-trekking through the western Pamir Mountain range at near 11,000 ft above sea level.

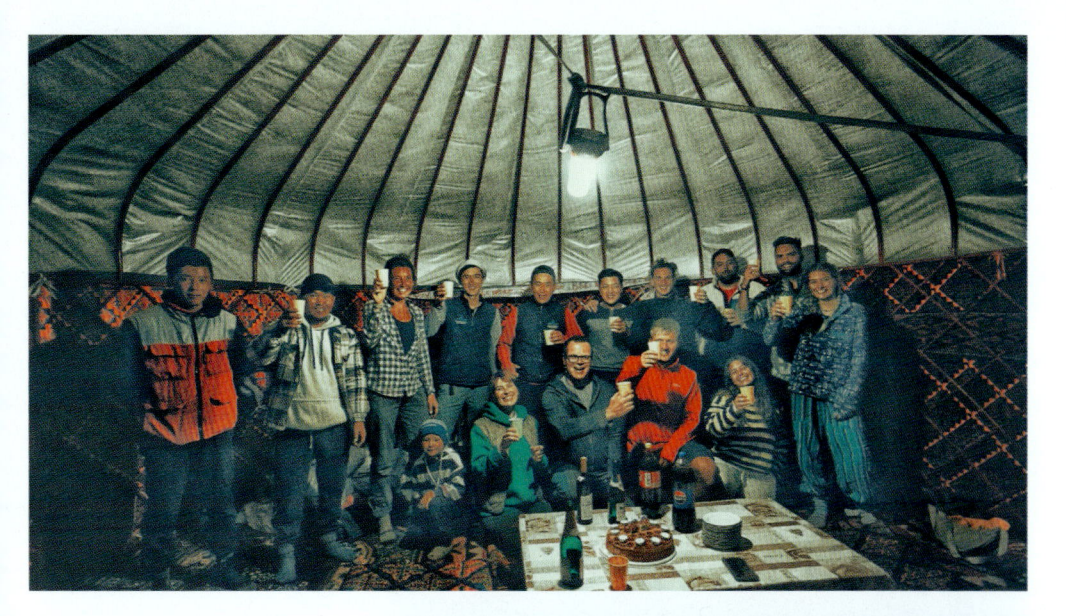

August 2024, Kyrgyzstan. Celebrating the first night with the horse-trek raffle competition winners, while being hosted by a nomadic family who fed us in their yurt.

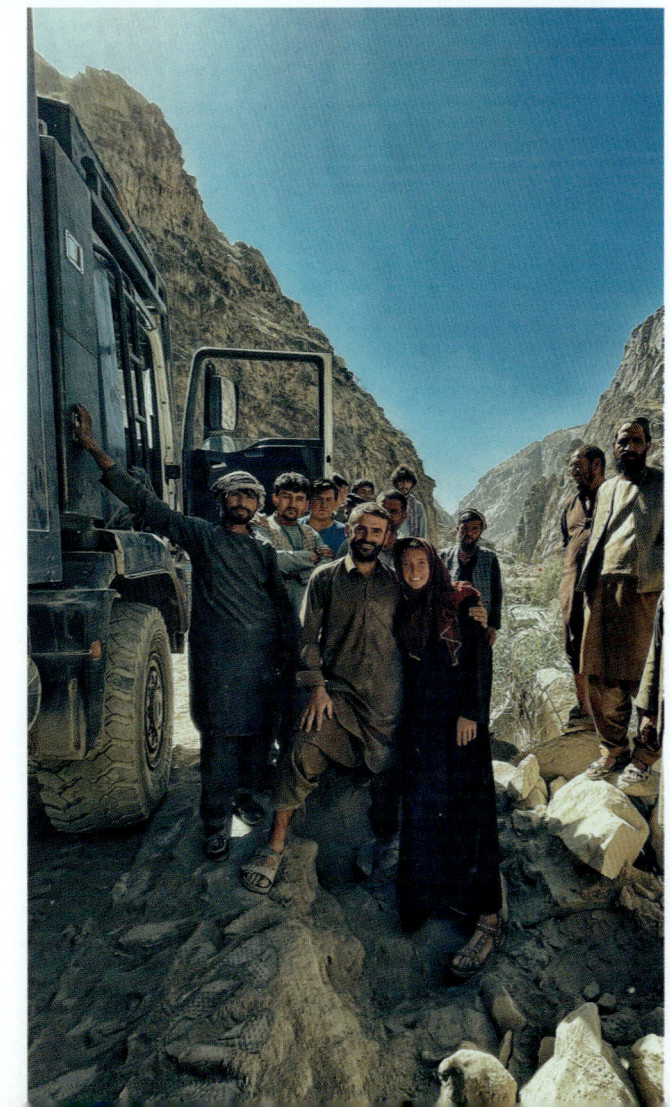

September 2024, Afghanistan. We take a snap with all the truck drivers at another unplanned stop, during our mammoth mountain diversion.

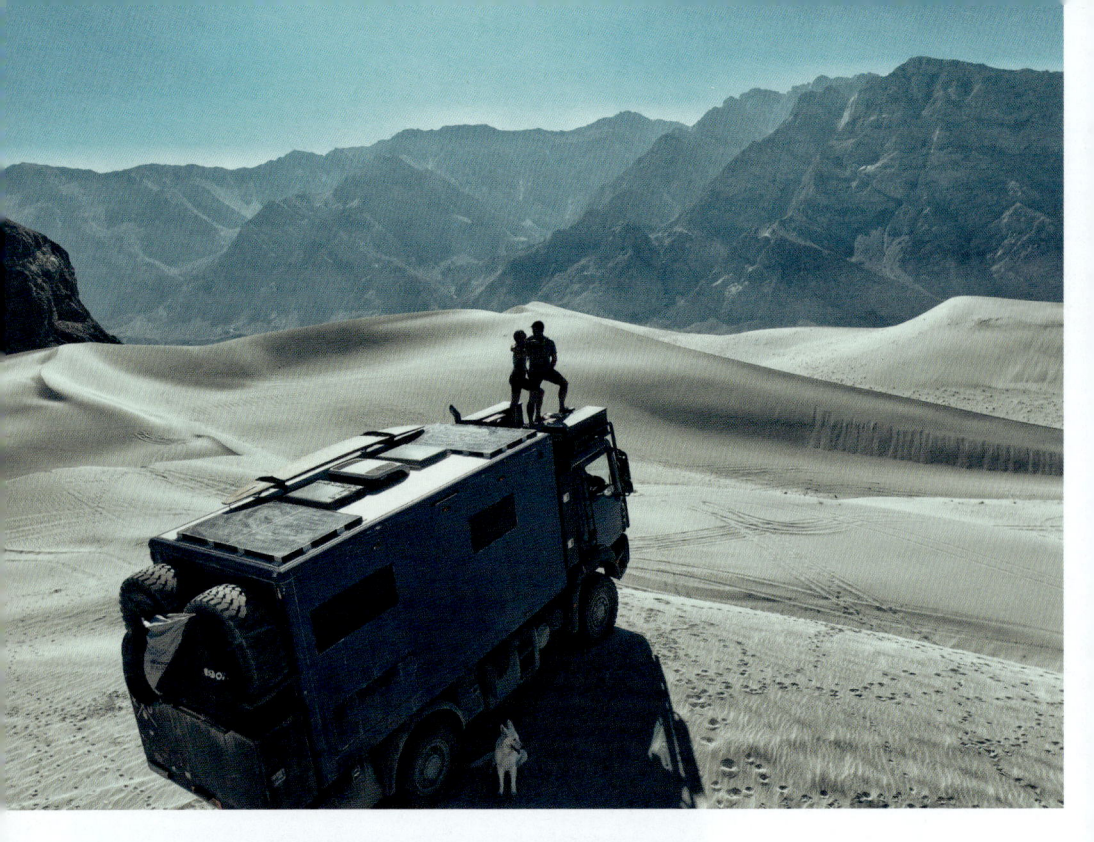

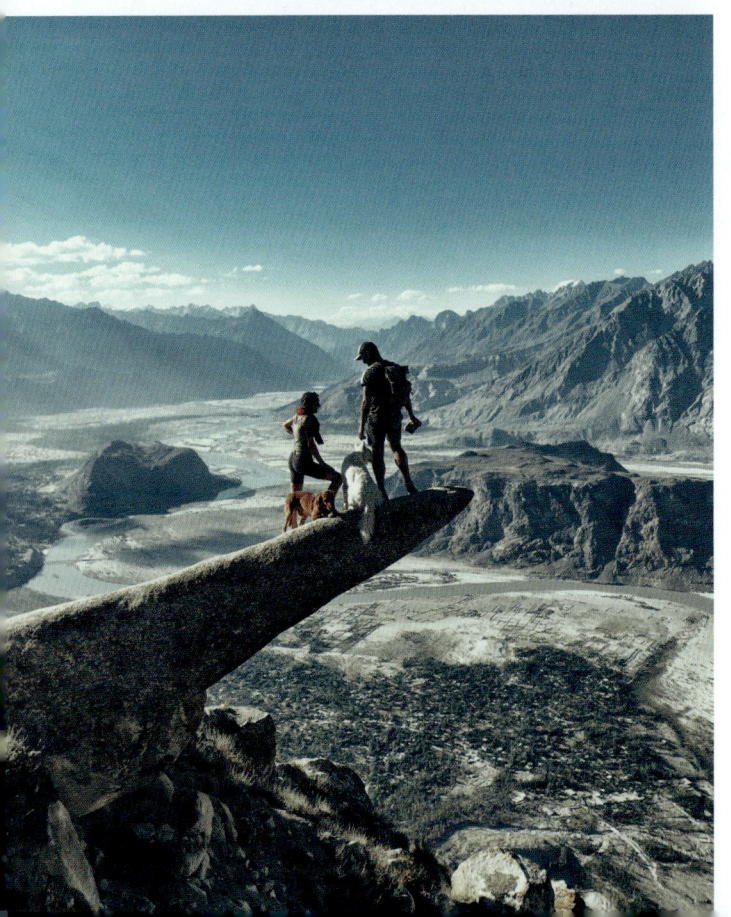

October 2024, Pakistan. The world's highest cold desert, the Katpana.

October 2024, Pakistan. Marsur Rock.

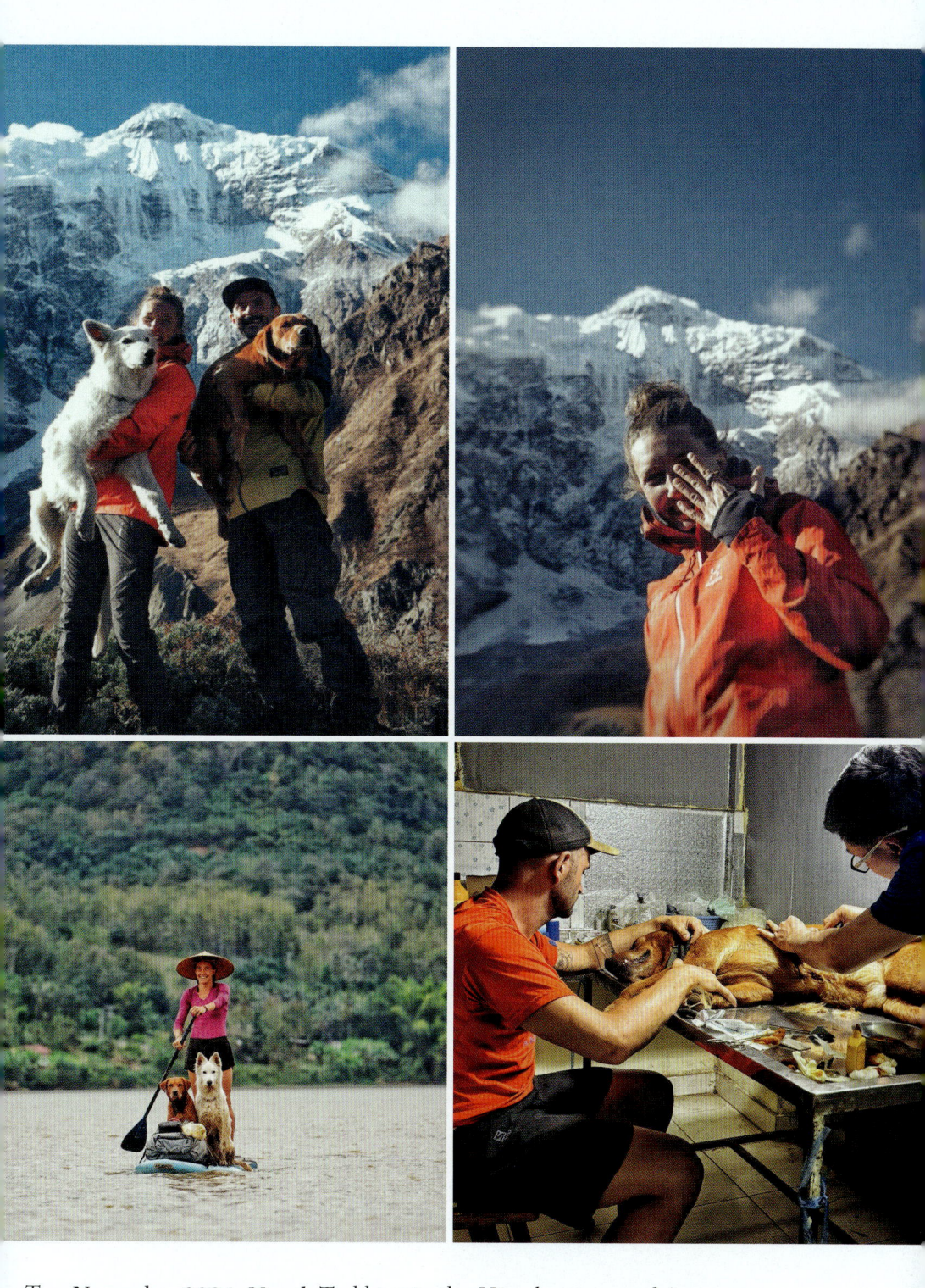

Top: **November 2024, Nepal.** Trekking in the Himalayas around Annapurna. The perfect spot to propose to Marie. *Bottom left:* **December 2024, Laos.** Paddleboarding down the Mekong River. *Bottom right:* **January 2025, Laos.** At the DIY vet, getting Red's stomach sewn up with fifteen stitches.

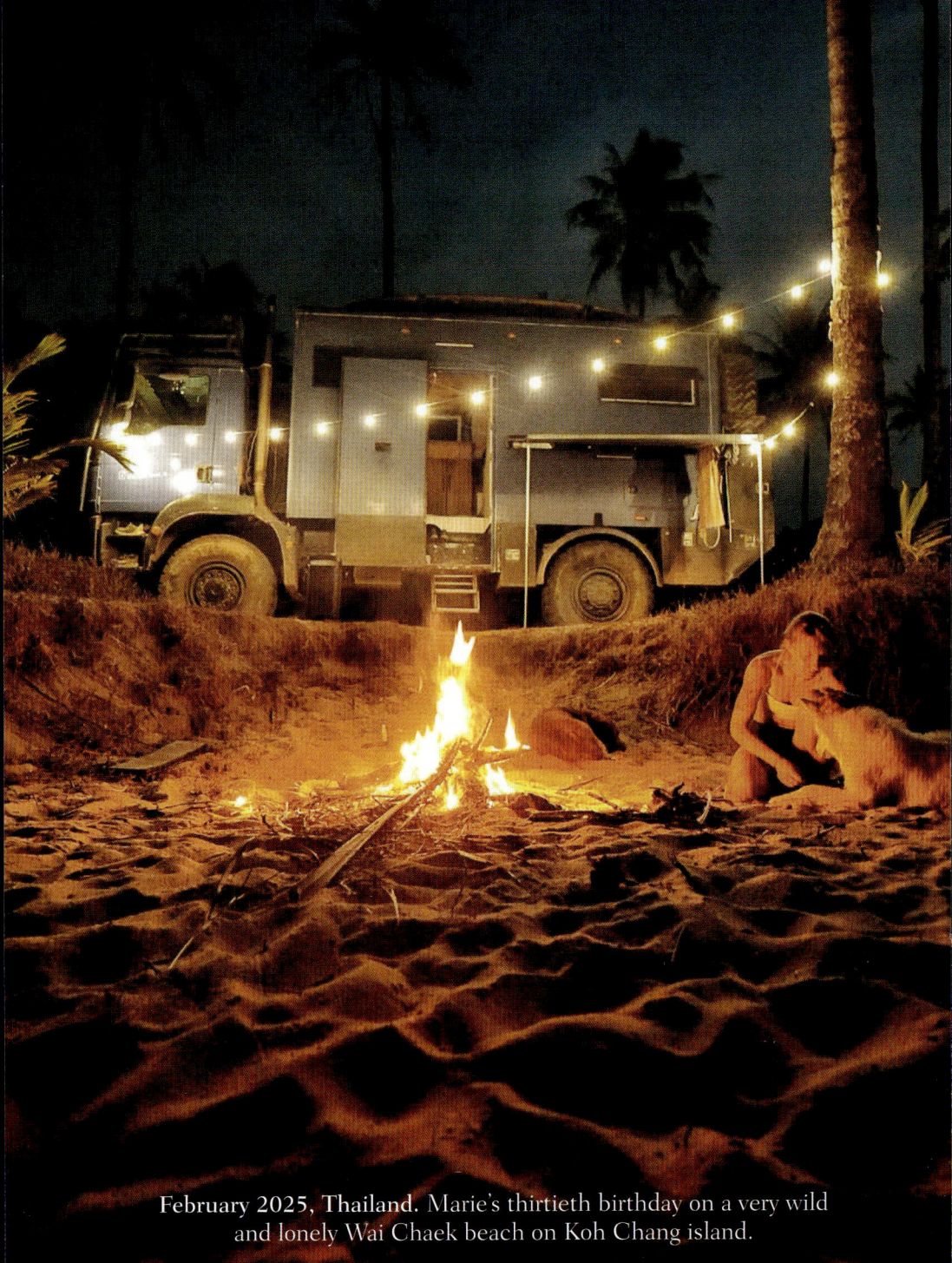

February 2025, Thailand. Marie's thirtieth birthday on a very wild and lonely Wai Chaek beach on Koh Chang island.

driving days. In silence, with Marie still shining her torch under the back, trying to figure out what was what, as I had run dry of any enthusiasm to explain what had happened, I stood up and slowly walked off towards the river's edge for a moment.

I was annoyed at myself for being so stupid, annoyed I'd come down the track unnecessarily, and feared what was to come. I'd done it once before, but this time, the ground was even boggier. There was no hope of using the hand winch, and whereas last time I was filled with adrenaline to fuel me to crack on, this time I just wanted to have a good sob.

A shoeless Marie came squelching down through the muddy grass.

'Come on, it'll be alright. We can do this. I've already got the spades out.'

I laughed a despairing laugh and shook my head.

'Thanks,' I said, leaning into her as she squatted down next to me.

'Wait, why have you got no shoes on?' I said, surprised enough to make myself chuckle.

'I didn't want to get my trainers or boots dirty,' she said, completely matter-of-fact in return.

I chuckled some more, shook my head, rose to my feet. 'Come on, you need to get some boots on. We can't rescue a truck from this bog, AND sew your toe back on after you've cut it off with the spade,' I said, laughing as my mood picked up.

I slowly got changed, moved things out of the way inside, knowing what a muddy bomb site the inside of the truck was about to become, all while letting out the odd swear word as memories from the night recovery in Italy came flooding back.

I stuck the speaker out of the door just as 9.04 p.m. appeared on my phone, put on a loud playlist of dance music I had made to motivate me before rugby games, and handed Marie a jam sandwich.

For the next two hours, we dug and cut our way under the back of the truck before Marie retrieved the jack and handed me all the kit, as I was now wedged under the back of the chassis in a cave made of metal. Those few hours will forever be the hardest and most demoralizing of my life. There wasn't enough space under the back to sit upright. I was leant against sharp brackets, which started to cut my chest, while I kept banging my head on the overhead rear air tanks. The truck was so low to the floor that despite attempting to dig using a normal-size spade, there wasn't enough room. I attempted to start jacking the truck, but I could only fit it on metal chassis sections. That meant that all I was able to achieve in an hour was to lift the truck up and down thirty centimetres on its suspension travel, without moving the wheel an inch. The only option was to dig lower, but thick roots ran underneath the only place I could use for jacking.

In desperation, Marie handed me our sharpest cooking knife and hammer, so while laying on my belly, wet through and in almost total darkness, I hammered the top of the knife into the roots and dug into the mud like some sort of crazed murderer.

At 1.09 a.m., I called it a day. Marie had been an absolute hero and without boots or losing a toe had cleared around

Truck It!

each of the wheels and loosely set two recovery boards. She had been grafting without a break or lodging a single complaint for four straight hours in awful conditions.

'This is now tomorrow's problem. It's stable enough so it's not going to sink. Let's get some rest.'

We both stripped naked on the steps outside the truck, and in the cold of the night, took an outside shower to clean ourselves.

The next morning at 7 a.m., after breaking out the emergency baked beans my nan had donated before I'd left, we got back to it.

'More beans,' I called for. 'More, honestly we are going to need it, Marie.'

I had been marching around outside, coffee in hand, assessing the scene of devastation surrounding the truck.

Coffees necked, food scoffed, we screamed and swore our way back into the cold, wet and muddy clothes from the night before.

For the final few hours, with motivation lifting as each wheel also lifted out of the quagmire, Marie set about propping stones and blocks of wood under the wheels, as I continued to man the jack.

'Bobby, I can't,' Marie struggled to say, lying on her front in the mud, both arms deep in the cold water surrounding the tyres, up to her armpits. 'Can you help hold this block down? It keeps wanting to float.'

I left the jack, laid down next to my girlfriend who was caked in mud, and stuck both arms into the murky water next to her to help. We both grunted with exertion as we moved stones and blocks around. Suddenly, I felt Marie's hands and I stopped to gently hold one of hers underwater in a romantic way. 'Isn't this cute,' I said. We both lay there laughing at the ridiculousness of the situation. Finally we managed to get enough blocks under the wheels to drive up and out of the field. We were freezing cold and utterly exhausted but elated.

'I'm starting to think we should get a proper winch,' I said.

The next morning, with the alarm set for 5 a.m., we drove to the border in silence in anticipation of what was to come. Both of us were nervous. We were about to enter a country at war – one that both our countries were very firmly supporting the other side in. This was a country that the official advice from both our governments was not to visit.

We came around the final corner and saw the Russian flag wafting large and menacingly in the June early morning light, high above the border post. I took a deep breath and turned in.

14

Russian Rushing

'Bobby, I think he's waving at us to stop!' shouted Marie.

Part of me thought about carrying on, but instead I slowed down, indicated and pulled over. I took a deep breath as I stepped out of the truck and walked towards the two policemen who stood a few feet away, with machine guns over their chests, staring at me.

'Hello!' I said, putting my big stupid tourist smile on. It helped people in authority feel more powerful and had often got us out of some sticky situations before, but I had a feeling it wasn't going to work here.

'Hello,' the Russian police officer said, shaking my hand in a firm but relaxed way. If George Clooney had a baby with a bear, he would look like this guy: handsome, tanned, with bright white teeth – but enormous.

'My friend,' he said, walking over and tapping the windscreen with the massive wooden club that had appeared in his hand. 'Is no good. Number illegal.'

The reg plate was slotted on the dashboard behind the window, still completely visible, but not actually on the front of the truck. Because that's where our shiny new winch was. *Bugger.*

Crossing Russia's border had involved a long queue before arriving in front of a woman who looked and sounded like a Bond villain. She shouted some Russian at us and gestured, at which point they opened a whole new lane for us, which was either a good or a very bad thing. We knew our cards wouldn't work in Russia and we decided against changing money, reasoning that we were going to be driving straight through and didn't want to stop. We'd filled the tank with fuel and fridges with food. 'Operation Sneak Through Russia' was about to commence.

We hopped out, both with sweaty palms, and were whistled like dogs towards a well-dressed guy as he disappeared through a door and into a booth marked 'Police'.

'Passport,' he said, holding out a hand. 'Hmmm, French,' he said, followed by an elated 'Great Britannia!!' and then something else in Russian.

Oh dear, I thought, trying to look calm.

A few guys walked over, cooing and opening our passports and looking at us, before losing interest and walking back to inspect the truck.

'Well, welcome to Russia,' the police inspector said in almost perfect English. My eyes opened as wide as saucers. 'How long do you intend on staying for?'

Truck It!

I couldn't get my words out. This smartly dressed guy, of similar age, had completely caught me off guard. *When was the interrogation going to start?* I thought.

'Three days only. We have a transit visa. Your English is fantastic!' I said back sheepishly.

'Aaaa yes, thank you. I am currently reading this novel by George Orwell,' he replied, lifting out an English copy of *1984* from behind his computer screen. 'Well, I hope you have a nice time here. I'm sorry you won't have more time to see our beautiful country,' he concluded, before he stamped our passports, stood up and barked orders at men hanging around the truck.

'Open. Open door. Inspection,' said a wiry-looking Russian soldier. He was evidently the main point man as others opened lockers, climbed on the roof and stood in the door of the cab, nervously wanting to get in as the dogs stared back at them.

'You don't have any rubles,' said another guard in perfect English, nodding at our display of bank notes from around the world, which we had pinned up on the roof of the cab. He had a big grin on his face as he fussed over Rubia. *Here we go*, I thought. *The shakedown.*

'No,' I said nervously. 'I'm afraid we didn't get chance to get any.'

'That is a shame,' he said smiling. 'Here.' And he reached into his pocket, pulled out his wallet, and took out a 100 ruble note. Taking some spare pins off the adjacent bank notes, he then pinned it next to one from Georgia.

'A present from Russia,' he said proudly as I chuckled in disbelief.

At what point do we get kidnapped and interrogated? I thought again as I climbed out of the cab and caught Marie laughing to something out of sight behind the truck.

'What's going on?' I said as I approached.

An elderly couple were walking off, waving to Marie. 'Welcome to Russia!' they shouted.

They'd left their car, which was being inspected in the next bay along, and walked over with a Russian sticker to add to our growing collection of flags on the back of the truck.

'I think they are Christians and wanted to wish us luck. That soldier cleaned a bit of the back and stuck it on for us,' said Marie. A nearby guy in uniform waved at me, smiling.

This wasn't what I was expecting. The customs paperwork was an interesting process as you filled in a form entirely in Russian, then threw it to three extremely angry women in a booth surrounded by a restless mob, who then slammed their shutter down and disappeared for five minutes. The form, with no other feedback bar red pen crosses, was then thrown back out randomly to the mob, who passed it between themselves to work out who had been rejected. After two hours, a Ukrainian guy took pity on us and helped Marie translate the form.

Paperwork completed and the offer to join the soldier who had gifted us the ruble note to eat dinner with his family that evening politely turned down, we set out from the border post.

'What do we put in the satnav? Kazakhstan?' I laughed in Marie's direction as this slapdash adventure felt like it had been elevated to the next level of craziness.

Truck It!

We made it about two hours before we met Clooney the bear.

'No, this is fine, completely normal. In my country this is legal. I have it registered like this,' I tried to blag, maintaining a straight face as he held his belly and laughed a big belly laugh.

'My friend, this is Russia. You must pay,' he said, looking deep into my soul. I realized I wasn't going to be able to mess with this guy.

'We will fix this now,' I said, deploying option two, before proceeding to use some zip ties to tie it awkwardly to the grille above the winch.

'There. Fixed. Sorry about that, sir, thank you.'

He held his hand up to stop me.

'My friend,' he said, still smiling brightly. 'You broke the law. This is no good. You must pay or go to jail. One hundred dollar or jail for three weeks,' he said.

I knew he was blagging, but we didn't have any time to waste. We had to get through before our visa expired. I also didn't fancy calling his bluff and visiting a rural Russian police station.

'I'm not sure we have the money,' I said, which set him off laughing again.

'Pay now,' he insisted, at which point the laughing abruptly stopped.

I jumped in the back, going for our stash of cash, as Marie followed me in.

A few stressful moments later and I jumped out: 'Fifty dollars,' I said, waving a note in his direction. 'That's all we have.'

'Wow,' he barked, looking around, clearly not liking the idea of being caught taking bribes off innocent tourists. 'Come.'

He ushered me to his police car, parked adjacent to the truck.

'I'm sorry for this, my friend,' he said, looking the least sorry I've ever seen someone look. 'But next time you will know.'

He coyly opened the glove box to reveal another stack of mixed notes from all around the world. 'Put money there,' he said as he looked out through the windows to check no one was watching.

I reached into my pocket, pulled out the ten-euro note I had retrieved from the truck, and quickly slipped it among the stack.

A grin appeared on his face, which set me off grinning too, which I had to fight to control.

'I'm so sorry,' I said, trying to remain as polite as I could. 'Thank you for making us feel safe, goodbye.'

'You didn't!' said Marie a few moments later when I told her what I'd done. 'Bobby!'

'Yeah, I did. I would have given him a fiver, if I had one. Good job he didn't check. That was the only gamble I knew I was taking.' I giggled in relief. Marie smirked and shook her head.

Russia is an absolutely enormous, incredibly varied country stretching over eleven time zones and comprising huge forests, rivers, lakes, mountains and cities full of incredible architecture from all throughout its rich history. Unfortunately, we didn't see any of that. Instead, seventy-two hours of

Truck It!

featureless driving later, and as the deadline loomed, we were a few hours out from the border before we started seeing more and more cars with nets that looked like tights over the whole front end. These weren't DIY things, either – these were custom-made, properly fitted . . . things.

'What on earth is that for?' I said inquisitively as we drove, spotting more and more appear.

'Fly nets, I think,' said Marie, squinting.

It was getting a bit swampy as we drove. It was 38°C (100°F), which, given we didn't have air con in the cab, meant we were driving with the windows down. Now, I don't know if you've ever encountered midges. They're pretty much everywhere, but particularly bad in Scotland. You might even have had a hike or a picnic ruined by them. But nothing – and I mean nothing – prepared me for what happened next.

Suddenly there were millions of them, and it was like driving through something solid. They covered everything – cars, houses, cattle; anything that gave off heat or breath. If you tried to breathe, you would inhale mouthfuls of them. They started Kamikaze-ing into my eyes and setting up refugee camps in my ears. I now understood why all the locals were walking around in huge hats with nets hanging from them, tucked neatly around their necks. Some wore gloves, others full-body suits, like bee keepers.

How anyone actually lived here was beyond me. We decided the only thing to do was to drive fast enough that the wind would blow most of them away. But then we hit the border queue and had to slow down. We shut the windows, but within minutes it was so hot in the cab we just had to open them again before either us or the dogs passed out.

'*Merde!* I can't stand thissss!' roared Marie half an hour later as she tried to wrap a shawl around her face, teaming it with a pair of sunglasses. She jumped out, called the dogs and all three of them got in the back and I heard the air con fire up. Smart. I, however, needed to keep shuffling the truck forward, so remained under attack.

'I know!' I called out. 'Wind!'

I scrambled to the tool locker, lay underneath the truck, connected the airline and blower attachment, stood back up and began blowing myself in the face like a hairdryer.

The car queuing behind us, windows up, air con blasting, looked at me like I'd lost it. I looked smugly back at them. The flying power of the midges couldn't cope with the airline's power, and the momentary relief was massive. Winner.

Five minutes later I got bored and went walking up and down the other empty lane of the road, whacking my face and head with a tea towel that Marie had passed me until it was time to inch forwards. If someone had designed a punishment in hell to annoy me, this would have been hard to beat.

Two excruciating hours later, as the barrier into the border post was only three cars ahead of us, something caught my eye in the wing mirror. I looked more closely and saw a car slowly queue-jumping, stopping to apparently talk to each driver. As he approached, I saw him wind his window down and chat with the driver behind us. The driver behind clearly wasn't happy. He waved his hands and dismissed him before winding his window back up.

Truck It!

'Little bastard,' I said, clocking what he was doing. 'He's trying to talk his way into skipping the queue,' I said to Marie, who had reappeared in hell next to me.

As the queue shuffled forward with the guy still behind us, I made sure to leave about ten millimetres of space in front of us. The car who had just been subject to his negotiations did the same as he tried to force his way in. The car stayed strong, not wavering from his line, almost touching bumpers, before the queue-jumper gave up and started approaching us.

There was no way I was letting this bastard push in. But Mr Queue-Jumper didn't try chatting to us, presumably recognizing that we were tourists, so went for the guy in front.

Thankfully, he too dismissed him, but, unlike the driver behind us, wasn't too keen to drive bumper to bumper in his nice new car. So, as we next edged forward and came to a halt, the queue-jumper had got half a nose in front.

The next thing I knew, I had jumped straight out of the cab from the top step, and was stomping towards the queue-jumper. Which, I'll be honest, surprised me as well.

'No! No! No way!' I shouted, followed by some profanities. 'We have been queuing here for hours and you think you can just come down here and push in. Not happening, mate!' I had completely lost it. We had been sat in hell for what seemed like an eternity, sweating and under constant attack. The temperature was pushing 40°C and I had snapped.

He wound down his window and started to say something calmly back to me, but I wasn't in the mood for negotiating.

'No, no way, I don't care. What makes you so special?! Go

back!' I shouted, waving my arms violently in his direction, turning my back on him to walk back to the truck.

'Come here,' said a deep voice from behind moments later, to which I swung round to see a bearded guy erupting from a small car, like a character from *The Lord of the Rings*, minus the sword and shield.

Had I seen the size of this fella prior to telling him to 'F off', I'm not sure I would have delivered the message with such vigour. Nonetheless, I had played a lot of rugby and could hold my own against much bigger guys, so I walked towards him, ready to let him have it again, when before I had chance to open my mouth, he punched me in the neck.

He had caught me completely off guard, but, being used to plenty of violence wearing short shorts on Saturday afternoons, I only took a few steps back before striding towards him ready to get stuck in.

Shoves turned into grappling and shouting, but he seemed to be a little taken aback by a guy who stood eight inches shorter, and weighing significantly less, putting up a fight.

Before it got out of hand, we were separated by onlooking truck drivers.

I looked over to see Marie, who was just shaking her head like a disappointed mother.

He was continuing to talk away in his language and I was shouting back at him. Then we both took a breath.

'Where are you from?' I asked.

'Azerbaijan,' he said grumpily.

'England,' I said.

Then, in the most ridiculous of moments, we both started furiously typing away on our translation apps. He read, then

Truck It!

typed a long response, which was a long garbled series of reasons why I was the one in the wrong and vice versa. After a few minutes, I started to see the funny side of things and the momentum dropped.

Our silent argument was interrupted before it could reach a conclusion as the queue began to move and we both quicky scurried back into our vehicles.

'Happy now?' said Marie, narrowing her eyes at me.

'Big bastard, wasn't he?' I said, laughing. 'I wasn't expecting that.'

Twenty minutes later we were stamped out of Russia, much to our relief, and got waved out. The big bastard stood arguing with a guard, so I took my chance to be the bigger man, hypothetically, and went up to him to shake his hand.

'Sorry, mate,' I said, 'good luck,' and winked at him.

I walked back to the truck with my chest puffed out like a pigeon.

'Big guy, terrible handshake,' I said to Marie, starting the engine.

My alpha maleness was only undermined slightly when, after driving through the miles of no man's land at the border, I started shrieking with excitement to Marie.

'Look, Marie, look! Camels!'

We had entered Kazakhstan.

15

Stanning the Stans

'He's having us on,' I declared confidently to Marie, who was sheltering in the shade from the vicious heat.

'What's he doing?' she asked, gently, so as not to get any hotter.

'He's in there with a stethoscope, listening to the fridge while he taps it.' I sat down on the hot ground. 'That was after he went at it with the grinder. Then he says he's going to take it for a bath.'

'You did say to do whatever it needed,' laughed Marie.

It turned out that the end of June in Uzbekistan was really different to the end of May in Georgia. Fewer avalanches for a start, but if we needed any clearer indication that we had completely left Europe behind us, the past three days since crossing the Russian border into Kazakhstan had

Truck It!

provided it. I may have never been to Georgia before, but the architecture, the wet, cool climate, the environment – it all felt familiar. And Russia had been one long sprint, which we'd spent almost entirely in the truck.

But now, as we set foot in central Asia, green grass had given way to white sand, and the cool mountain breeze was replaced by oven-hot, dry air.

As soon as we'd got into Kazakhstan from Russia, we had exchanged money on the border with a toothless woman, still wearing a big midges net (though they had begun to thin out). Then we sorted insurance from a guy in a plywood hut with a bunk bed at the back and a shoulder-level desk in the front.

It was a thankless task trying to translate the information he needed for what we all knew was a completely useless piece of paper, but we soldiered through, handed over the cash and hit the open road.

I decided that Russia had been so full-on, we deserved a break, so aimed the truck towards a lake. Or so I thought. It was only as we were approaching it that I realized it was the Caspian Sea. The problem was, we couldn't seem to find it.

We wound our way along sandy tracks around dunes before we passed what felt like a beach and shoreline. Out of the window, Marie pointed at a 'no swimming' sign jutting up out of the sand.

'That's weird.'

I pulled up Google Earth, and according to that, we had not only found the Caspian Sea; we were in it.

I realized that over to the other side of us were the remains of a beached fishing boat. We decided to see how far it had receded and it was about half a mile before we hit water. Later, I would read that climate change, exacerbated by the number of dams along the Volga river in Russia, meant that in some places the coast had receded by as much as twenty kilometres.

'This is absolutely nuts,' I said. 'This is what we were meant to cross under the original plan if Azerbaijan's borders were still open,' I explained. 'There's a ferry you could take from Azerbaijan to Kazakhstan, which cuts out either Russia or Iran.'

So, after a well-earned sandy day of rest surrounded by herds of wild camels, we once again set the compass east and decided to make a beeline for the Uzbekistan border, only a day's drive away across barren, featureless desert steppes. The horizon was broken only by a never-ending row of power lines and the odd dollop of camel dung.

We had been warned that the border between Kazakhstan and Uzbekistan would be a difficult one and we should expect a full strip search of the truck, so we made sure the drone was well hidden, since they are banned in Uzbekistan.

It felt bad to lie to our new friend the border guard who helped us navigate the paperwork as six very serious-faced border officers swarmed the truck, checking every little nook and cranny. I didn't think I suffered from anxiety until the guards started removing the kitchen drawers and checking the label of each box of medicine Marie had brought along with her. Then I almost had a panic attack inside as Marie swanned around outside taking selfies with the other border guards and the dogs.

Truck It!

A few sweaty hours later and we were back driving through almost identical desert. Some borders, you can really feel the difference either side. This one, not so much. That was, until we got talking to an exhausted-looking Czech family at a remote border post.

'These roads are truly the worst we have driven,' they said, pointing back the way they had come and shaking their heads as their two gloriously feral kids ran around like crazy. I caught Marie watching them and smiling. We had talked about how it seemed like you had to pick a life of adventure *or* kids. This trip, I had presumed, was a drive with a destination and an end point, where I hoped I would rediscover my purpose like a pot of gold at the end of a rainbow. And yet, here we were chatting to a wild family full of crazy tales, raising their kids on the road.

I looked back at their parents, who had wild eyes and scruffy hair, and it brought back the moment I first set my sights on that family in the old Land Rover who had sparked the dream while I stood outside the pub.

Maybe, I thought.

'For perhaps sixty miles, it is very bad, then the tarmac turns to dirt tracks, which are better.'

I thought they must have got the English wrong, until we got to the 'road'.

Fair play to them. The tarmac was more like concrete and littered with what I can only describe as bomb craters, some of them five feet wide and waist-deep. We watched as a line of huge trucks coming out from the horizon threw up dust clouds as they wove in a majestic pattern to avoid them.

'This is ridiculous,' I said to Marie after twenty minutes

of fighting with the steering wheel. 'I can't keep any sort of speed and you can't even see the bloody things to judge if they are little shallow ones or will break the truck in two. Let's try over there.' I pointed to the car tracks in the sand that ran adjacent to the road, weaving around the dunes. I turned off and got stuck in.

'Whooooooo! I feel like a rally driver!' I called as we flew along the track at almost fifty miles an hour, weaving around and over sandy obstacles, soon overtaking the trucks on the concrete track to our right. The further east we got, the more the sand turned to dust. A huge cloud dragged behind us for twenty metres. It was like something out of *Mad Max*. It was when we stopped for water after an hour that Marie discovered the disaster scene.

The fridge, already loosened from off-roading in the mountains of Albania, had given up entirely and ejected onto the floor of the truck, spilling its contents everywhere, including a massive amount of our drinking water. We picked up as much food as we could and crossed our fingers as we screwed the fridge back into place. Not having a fridge in this forty-degree heat would make things very tricky indeed, with roadside food shacks being very sparse. An hour later and our fears were confirmed. It was kaput.

After three days driving as fast as one can over sand in a ten-tonne truck, we erupted out of the desert like Lawrence of Arabia into an oasis town.

We were so dehydrated from crossing the first 'steppe', we crawled into the nearest shop and I drank 1.5 litres of fresh juice in one sitting, stopping only twice to gasp for air. Then we gorged ourselves on the utterly delicious pastries full of

Truck It!

meat called *samsa*. And, to finish, the sweetest watermelon you've ever tasted in your life. Honestly, heaven is an Uzbek watermelon.

The dogs were suffering in the heat as well. We were bouncing them between the cab and the back with the air con running as the temperature peaked around midday. The hot dry wind was incessant. It was like being in a fan oven. We had also given up on them sleeping inside the truck for the heat, so were now setting up their beds outside on the floor under the truck, to give them room to breathe. There was no let-up at night, as it was still 33°C. So, once we loaded up on drinking water, we set out to find someone to give the fridge the kiss of life.

'Okay, finish,' the now shirtless sixty-year-old man declared, stumbling out of his workshop in flip-flops and shorts, sweating from wrestling with the fridge. It was 11.30 p.m.

I laughed, raised my eyebrows and cocked my head, not quite believing it. The past few hours had seen the whole back of the fridge missing in some sort of pipes and wires open-heart surgery, before more grinding took place, more men were called and, yes, it was given a bath.

Then a big Russian guy appeared, hugging the fridge, marching towards the truck.

He took two big steps up, held it in place, and slotted it in, as if it were as big as a shoe box.

Twenty minutes of chatting later, during which a young woman approached Marie to give her earrings as a gift, followed by a flag of the autonomous region we were in, Karakalpakstan, and the fridge began to run cold.

'Wow, I'm very impressed,' I said simply. 'How much?' I

asked, rubbing my thumb and finger together, knowing that four guys had spent the best part of all day on it.

'For you, my friend, fifty dollars,' he replied.

'Deal,' I said, shaking his hand. Which it was. The fridge cost a little over a thousand pounds back in the UK and ran uniquely on 24v. Getting a replacement out here – in fact, getting a replacement before reaching Australia – would be impossible. We had been extremely lucky to find these guys, who were air con specialists and agreed to 'have a go' at the fridge repair.

After the desert crossing and fridge drama, it was an incredible relief to reach a river near the Turkmenistan border the next day and spend the afternoon with ten guys who had finished work early to get extremely drunk, eat an incredibly tasty barbecue and swim in the river. We had a great laugh with them. The next day we set off once again into the desert, keeping one eye on the fuel gauge given the country had little to no diesel since pretty much everything ran on liquid petroleum gas.

Two days later, I was forced to admit defeat. We had stopped to fill up our drinking water at the side of a road from a public fountain, without stopping to think where it had come from, and had eaten incredible-looking pastries at a roadside stall – the combination of which meant I was now stopping every twenty minutes to produce my own version of liquid petroleum gas. Being ill at home, as people fuss around you, is one thing. Driving along, shivering with stomach cramps, while sitting in a pool of your own sweat in forty-three-degree heat, is something else.

We were driving big days to try to escape the searing

heat, knowing the sanctuary of cooler mountain air lay just over Uzbekistan's eastern border with Kazakhstan, but we didn't make it before I gave up. We had driven more than 1,500 miles east and then south from the Caspian Sea and had picked up the old Silk Road route heading east, where once traders would have carried silk, spices, salt and furs. But now I was after only one thing, and it wasn't a woven product.

Hot and flustered, I stormed into one, two and then a third HGV and machinery shop just outside the historic town of Samarkand, before coming across an aftermarket air con unit. I was so relieved I could have skipped.

'How much?' I pointed.

He typed 400 dollars into the calculator, but honestly, he could have asked for a thousand and I would have said yes.

We settled at 350, knowing I'd had my pants down, but I wasn't for playing hard ball and shuffled back out into the sun, boxes in hand.

We set off in search of somewhere to start installing it ourselves and found a putrid field used as an informal rubbish dump, picked a corner upwind and began trying to sift through the box to find the Chinese instructions.

'Do you know what you're doing? Have you fitted one of these before?' asked Marie, who was once again ready to get stuck in.

'Nope. But it can't be rocket science. My motto is if "he" can do it, so can I. Can't be that hard.'

A few hours of stripping, drilling, wiring and replacing – followed by an expensive and very confusing trip to a car air con garage, where the mechanic was extremely confused to see a big truck arrive asking for a pipe on the roof to be connected – we had glorious ice-cold air.

'Noisy, isn't it?' Marie giggled as she held her palms up to cold air.

'What?' I shouted ironically to her as we laughed above the sound of the aeroplane jet engine to the side of our heads.

'Honestly, I don't care if I'm deaf, as long as I'm not sweating my bollocks off all day,' I screamed.

But even with the air conditioning, I was in a bad way. I was sweating so much, I was struggling to keep myself hydrated. And I'd lost a huge amount of weight. I was surviving on a diet of raw garlic, fresh carrot and honey. I felt so bad, I assumed I must have picked up a parasite. I was tired of driving, tired of borders, tired of feeling rough. I was exhausted and emotional and if someone had given me a button to press and I'd be magically 3,300 miles north-west, home at the pub with friends and family, I may well have pushed it.

Instead, I squeezed Marie's hand and kept the truck pointing at the distant dark of the mountains where the cool mountain air was the medicine I was in desperate need of.

16

Buzzing in Kyrgyzstan

'What is this?' demanded the stern Kyrgyzstan border guard.

My heart absolutely sank. I stumbled to come up with a response as he turned around with the vibrator in his hand.

'Ooh, er, I wouldn't,' I said and tried to grab it. 'Neck massager, neck massage. Brrrrrrrrr,' I said, and pretended to rub it down the back of my neck, trying to mime becoming relaxed from a massage. 'Aahhhh,' I said, now relaxed.

His younger colleague, a bloke of about my age, was having absolutely none of it and was laughing hysterically. This made his boss even more annoyed, who questioned him loudly as he tried to catch enough breath to explain to him. I tried to keep a straight face as I watched the older guy putting two and two together before putting the 'massager' down firmly on the side.

Marie, oblivious to what was happening at yet another border crossing, stood enjoying the early July sunshine on the other side of the checkpoint, chatting with a Polish hitchhiker.

The boss man held his scowl and continued to root around the truck.

'What's this?' he said, holding up our best cooking knife, stored in a leather sheath to keep it sharp.

'Cooking knife. To eat,' I said, making an eating mime.

'No. Illegal. Dangerous.' He leaned out of the truck, barked orders at the young guard who had wandered over to tell his mates about the sex toy they had just found. A minute later, the younger guy reappeared without any sign of a smile, passing a picture with a collage of banned items, one of which was a picture of a sheathed knife with a description of the legal amount of serration permitted.

'No. This is for cooking.' I opened the drawer where it was stored and threw around some knives, forks and spices to make my point.

'No. Illegal. Pay fine or jail,' he barked.

Not this again, I thought.

Back to plan B. As he marched out of the truck with the knife in hand to show everyone else and then reaffirm his point was correct, I hurried to the back of the truck, opened the locker and grabbed the grinder and grinding disc.

Without giving him the option, I approached the guy, who turned, looking confused.

I pulled the knife out of the sheath, leaving him holding it, half turned, so I wouldn't spray everyone at the border with sparks, and blunted the knife.

Truck It!

I then passed him back the knife, holding the blade to prove it was now not illegal or any more of a threat than a spoon, and proudly marched to the truck to put the grinder back.

'Pay fine,' he spluttered, handing the knife back, a shocked look on his face.

'No fine,' I replied, very matter-of-fact.

I walked back to the truck, threw the knife in the drawer, shut the door and started to climb the stairs into the cab.

'Finish, go now?' I half asked, half declared to the younger guy, as the boss man had lost interest and was walking off.

'Go,' he waved, annoyed at me.

I chuckled, started the truck and set off towards the gate that was opening in front of me.

Even though the change from the west of Kazakhstan to the east had been an incredible move from desert sand to green pastures and hills, we'd kept on pushing for the border. The first thing I did when we'd crossed back into East Kazakhstan was sleep for two days. As Marie played with the dogs in the clear mountain rivers, my body fought with and finally beat whatever had been wrong.

'All part of the story,' I said to Marie as I came out of the truck, bleary-eyed with sleep but feeling human again finally. She later confessed that for the first time this whole trip, she'd been really worried about me.

We drove down out of the wilderness and arrived into the city of Almaty. After so many days in the arid desert, it felt surreal to be in a city. Framed by the Trans-Ili Alatau mountains, it was full of parks and trees in between the office and housing blocks, and there were shops and restaurants everywhere. We parked up and got out, only to discover we were opposite a French boulangerie and an amazing Italian restaurant. Bingo. I took this as a sign that the universe was telling me I needed to eat pain au chocolate and pizza to regain all my lost weight within three hours.

Once my stomach cramps had settled down, this time from eating too much fantastic food, it was on to Charyn Canyon, where Charley Boorman and Ewan McGregor had ridden their motorbikes in *Long Way Round*, which had captivated me when I was ten years old. I knew I had to see it. However, in the past twenty-odd years, it had become completely swallowed in cafes and gift shops and you could no longer drive there like they had. Annoyed at myself for not checking first, I found a nearby lake on the map and decided we would explore the area for our final few days in Kazakhstan, before we crossed yet another border towards Kyrgyzstan.

The lake turned out to be one of the most beautiful places I had ever seen in my life. The clearest, bluest water, surrounded by deserted tracks used to service the high mountain shepherds. For three days, we bumped, slipped, revved and forced our way up and through canyons, over rivers and across plateaus before arriving on the moon. We had aimed for a hill that rose up like a stalagmite in the middle of a vast valley. When we reached the top, it was as if a helicopter had dropped us off. There was no one in sight for miles and miles, only the odd herd of goats or chamois in the far distance. That night we lay and looked up at the brightest stars we had seen on the trip, with dogs for pillows. We both lay in silence, lost in our own thoughts.

Truck It!

Our little honeymoon was only briefly interrupted for an impromptu five-hour fuel filter change, when a light saying STOP IMMEDIATELY started flashing red. We were twenty miles or more from the nearest actual road, in the middle of nowhere, with no phone signal. I guessed that the last lot of fuel we'd bought in Uzbekistan from a barrel had been full of crap and clogged the line. We swore, got covered in diesel and became mildly hysterical at one point as we couldn't find an important but delicate spring that had sprung off into long grass. But when we turned the ignition, silently praying as the truck spluttered and threw out thick grey smoke, it came to life.

Onwards we went, towards the next country: Kyrgyzstan. The whole place had been a mystery to me when I'd set out, other than my sister once telling me it was 'honestly really beautiful'. But that hadn't prepared me for what Switzerland must have looked like 200 years ago, before roads, ski resorts and hotels arrived. As summer got into full swing, we drove through enormous green valleys carpeted with pine forests, past crystal-clear lakes. It was as if the giant scale of our surroundings suddenly made more sense of the truck. Often, in Europe, we had felt too big for our surroundings, but among the mountains and nomads, fuel was cheap, roads were wide, and the scenery to die for. This was where the truck was built to roam.

We filled the truck with half a tonne of fresh water, piled the fridge to the brim and just pointed the truck at a mountain, knowing that, if we needed to, we could be self-sufficient for weeks. Away from the main roads and towns, horses were still the main way of getting around. When the winter snow melts and the mountain passes reopen, nomads pack their lives onto their trusty steeds and head deep into the mountains with their herds of cattle to allow them to graze on painted green hillsides. Over those weeks we would often try to get as far away as we could, driving and hiking into the middle of nowhere, only to find a nomadic horseman staring down at us from a distant ridgeline with their herd of cattle spread out on the hillside below.

How they survived and reached those places, I will never know.

The day we paddleboarded and camped in the wilderness is one I won't forget for a long time. There were no roads, or buildings, or electricity pylons. It was just mountains, water and sky. The same view that has been here for thousands of years. We glided along and the water was so clear that a second range of mountains stretched downwards below the mirror-like surface. Most of the time reflections are like shadows, just the shape but nothing more. But in these you could see detail, colour, individual clumps of vegetation. It was like someone had changed the settings on reality. There was no sound but our paddles dipping in and out of the water. It was so beautiful, we just grinned as we silently paddled along with the dogs sat on the front.

When my last relationship ended and my business hit hard times, it had felt like the end of the world. But now I can see they were like ropes holding down a hot-air balloon, and when cut, it could start to rise. And now here I was, rising up and out of the haze of depression into the blue sky of a new life, looking down at this beautiful world.

Truck It!

Birthdays were usually just another day, but, being on an adventure of a lifetime, it felt like the right excuse to make something of my thirty-second, so, in need of another fix of adventure, we decided to hike up to summit a 13,000ft mountain just south of Bishkek. The birthday plans almost fell through before we started, though, as an official-looking bloke approached and declared that no dogs were allowed up the valley.

'Bollocks,' I swore, throwing back down my heavy bags I'd just clipped up.

We decided to wing it and climb up a different hill slightly further down the valley, out of sight of Mr Killjoy. It was a hard slog straight up the hill carrying huge packs with more kit than we had originally planned, as it turned out we needed to sort our own accommodation and food for a couple of days, rather than stay in the climbers' mountain lodge just below the summit. We walked until it got dark, pitched our tent, exhausted, and fell immediately asleep.

Early the next morning, we woke to the sound of our dogs barking and whimpering, only to find we (I) had pitched our tent in a riverbed in the dark, which was now filling with freezing-cold run-off water from higher up the mountain. Having originally told them to bugger off and let me sleep, the dogs now had a 'help me' look about them.

Marie jumped straight up and ran out before I had time to come around. Thirty seconds later she came squelching back and started singing 'Happy Birthday' while holding out a tiny chocolate cake complete with two candles, just about still alight. I thought back to the number of birthdays I had worked through over the past decade.

'Marie, we are halfway up a mountain! How have you done that!' I laughed.

Then she produced a small box of chocolates.

'Ta daa!' she announced as I gratefully accepted my gift. 'They didn't have cards, so this will have to do.'

She handed me a neatly folded chunk of toilet roll, on which she had written a beautifully handwritten birthday message. I felt my eyes start to get a bit weepy. It was so kind, and I hadn't been expecting it at all. Especially not halfway up a lonely mountain in a soggy tent. It was still surprising to be reminded of just how low and lacking in confidence I had been when I'd met Marie. I realized how deep it had gone into the core of who I was. But, slowly, with every day we spent together, it was as if she was repairing my soul.

'I don't deserve this,' I said.

'Yes, you do,' she said.

17

Horsing Around in Kyrgyzstan

'Oh bugger. Marie, he's gone!'

I was wearing only my boxer shorts as the dogs sniffed around me, looking for the perfect place to do their morning wee.

'Bobby. Chill,' said Marie, calmly making coffee. 'He won't have gone far. Look, down there, he's probably just gone to say hello to his mates.'

The 'he' Marie was referring to was a beautiful brown horse, who we had nicknamed Hoppy. He had been entrusted to us by one of the horsemen, who had arrived and explained via the translation app that he needed to leave said horse here for the night and he would come and collect him in the morning, before hitching a lift on a passing beat-up old car and driving off down the dusty mountain track.

Bobby Bolton

'Well, I guess we're horse-sitting tonight,' I'd said.

It was another beautiful mountain morning in late August, and we were on the start of the Pamir Highway the second highest highway in the world, at over 4,500 metres. Tomorrow we would be crossing into Tajikistan. Well, we would if we could find this bloody horse.

It had been an incredible month in Kyrgyzstan since my birthday.

I had come limping down the mountain after twisting my knee after I'd been concentrating on my whistling, rather than the terrain under my feet, but there was no time to waste, as we were straight off to the airport at Osh, to pick up my dad. He had flown over to look after the truck and dogs while we took a whistle-stop, five-day trip back to the UK for my mate Max's wedding and for Marie to nip back and see her mum.

My dad arrived, said 'Hello' in his massive, booming Wigan voice, then proceeded to take photos of everything that seemed 'exotic' as we drove from the airport, which included road signs, tuk-tuks and a man driving cattle down the roadside. My dad hadn't visited anywhere outside of Europe before, so Kyrgyzstan may as well had been Mars to him.

We'd plotted a route for him to drive while we were away, and the plan was we'd all meet up again in five days' time. The fact that he immediately set off on the wrong side of the road didn't fill me with confidence, however.

'Please don't drive our home off a cliff, Mark,' called Marie.

Four days later, we were in the middle of the Yorkshire Dales when my phone went off. Dad. Half expecting bad

Truck It!

news, I took the call, only to realize I had a close-up video of my dad's ear.

'Everything okay, Dad?'

'Bobby!' I probably didn't even need the phone to hear him, he was always shouting so loud on the phone. 'Bobby, look! I've got new friends!'

He pulled the phone back to reveal an enormous family of mums, dads, grandmas and grandpas and loads of kids all cheering and waving.

'I went to the pool by the river and there was this family and they were playing with the dog and then we all had lunch and then they invited me to have dinner with them. I can't believe it!' Over the few days he was babysitting and having his own little slice of adventure, it was as if he'd made friends with the entire population of Kyrgyzstan, and about a hundred selfies started coming through.

'Bobby, I don't want to come home,' he said the last time I spoke to him before he got on his return flight. 'These dogs, this country, it's just . . .' he trailed off.

'I know exactly what you mean, Dad,' I said.

It was so surreal to have this tiny leap back home. After spending so much time with just the two of us, I kept catching Marie's eye, both overwhelmed by so many people asking thousands of questions. I didn't feel I'd done the best job of communicating to them what the trip so far had been like. I literally didn't have the words to do it justice.

'Bobby, you are so lucky,' whispered Adele, the bride, as a group of wedding guests all surrounded Marie to probe her.

Friends, family members, random guests and even the waiter in the pub all declared, rather sheepishly, that they were huge fans of what we were doing, and all pried for some inside gossip.

'What are the chances . . . it must have been fate . . . I can't believe how well you match . . . that black eye she got looked awful . . .'

It was the same all night as we bounced between groups to catch up and to introduce Marie. But introductions weren't really needed, since all of them spoke to us like they were Marie's best friend.

Travelling halfway round the world is like being in a bubble. We take ourselves from place to place, hitting record as often as we can, trying to describe, portray and demonstrate what an amazing adventure we are on. But bar the odd call back to a family member every now and then, there is never any tangible feedback. The follower count might be going up, but it was only being back here, surrounded by our closest friends, that we saw how much we had captivated the imagination of so many, all of whom dreamt of driving off into the sunset with us.

However, four whirlwind days later, we were back to our reality in the truck, setting off again up into the Pamir mountains. We were four hours off-road, following a river up from a shallow valley, where it had been wide and slow, to a small, steep stream. Then we came up over the crest of a hill onto a small plateau. We were trying to follow a track, up and over the mountain, where we could see there was a lake. However, surrounded on all sides by forest and steep cliffs, we called our plan off. We were 8,000ft up and needed some flat ground to sleep. Marie and I scouted about and saw that there were two yurt camps where a nomadic family were

Truck It!

living through the summer. We reasoned we needed to give both of them a polite distance and were trying to work out where that might be when Marie called out to me quietly: 'Bobby, there's a guy coming over.'

I walked around the truck to see what was happening.

'Come, food, please,' he beckoned us.

'Er, yeah, sure, thank you,' we said. Leaving the dogs tied up in the shade with some fresh water, we walked out to his camp, which was composed of some animal huts, a hut built crudely of trees felled by hand and hand-sawn to create a small shed, a small one-man tent and yurt. Dozens of horses, goats and cows grazed nearby in the emerald green mountain pastures.

A little girl, of seven or eight, who I assumed was his daughter, came to greet us riding a melancholy looking donkey, waving a little twig she was using as a whip.

'Please,' he said, gesturing towards the blanket that an older woman wearing a long dress and traditional headscarf was laying out. More women appeared from the hut, holding bread, butter, honey and a big pan of *plov*, the traditional sticky rice dish.

'We make,' he said, pointing at all the tasty food. I couldn't quite believe it.

'Really?' I enquired.

'Yes. Bees there,' our host confirmed, pointing to a cluster of hives. 'Mother, very good cook,' and he tapped his mum on the back, who came over all embarrassed.

I pointed at the meat in the stew and said, 'Moooooo?'

She laughed and shook her head – then gestured to two goats tied across the field.

'This is incredible,' I said to Marie as we both tucked in.

I could see myself living like this. I thought it funny how my perception of what the future could look like had changed so fast. Once, it had been full of aspirations for a nice car, a full bank account and expensive coffee. Now I was dreaming of a life of adventure, of being smelly, wild and unkempt, roaming the world from one beautiful, crazy place to another.

Marie watched the little girl with a smile on her face; she was too energetic to sit and eat, instead going to talk to the horses, then leading her donkey into the stream, shouting 'Ya, ya!', before going to usher the chicken back towards the camp.

'She's so cool,' Marie whispered to me. 'I want my daughter to be like her.'

We all giggled at the sight. 'Yeah, I agree,' I said.

There was no phone service, so no way to translate, which meant our conversations were very broken.

'Daughter mum,' he said, forgetting the name for wife and pointing back down the valley. 'Home, small baby.' He picked his phone up: 'No speak, no phone,' he said.

Which gave me an idea.

I jogged back to the truck and returned with a bowl of chocolate and a nifty bit of kit my dad had brought with him – a mobile satellite dish called Starlink. (At this point, Elon Musk was yet to double the price of it overnight, so we could still use it.) I held up my phone and pointed at the Wi-Fi symbol as his eyes lit up. Two minutes later, his wife was holding up a tiny baby and speaking excitedly.

'I have not spoken to her for three months,' he typed on

the now functioning translation app, looking slightly emotional as he did so.

The rest of the family scrambled to find and switch on their phones. Soon there were five conversations as they caught up with their friends and family across the valley.

An hour later, as we fussed about in the stream washing clothes, a small group of nomadic people had amassed a polite distance away from the truck on a couple of fallen trees.

'For you. Please use,' I said. I couldn't help but feel that Wi-Fi was a less human gift than bread and honey, but seeing the joy in everyone's faces as they got in touch with their loved ones, it felt like a small way to repay their generosity and kindness.

That evening, they invited us for dinner, where again there was an incredible array of food. Through the phone translator, we found out that our host was a national champion in the Kyrgyzstan national sport of Kok-Boru, a brutal game best described as rugby meets polo, in which horsemen wrestle a dead sheep across a line.

'Please,' he said, handing me his Kok-Boru whip.

'I can't,' I said. 'Too special.'

But he kept his head bowed and continued to hold it out to me. 'Please,' he said.

Later he showed me how he would hold it in his mouth during the match; he played me a video of him crossing the goal line, reins in one hand, dead sheep in the other, and whip in his mouth.

We said goodbye the next morning and headed up to a different peak. That night, at about 10,000ft above sea level, we sat in silence watching the sun lower behind the mountains as the dogs napped at our feet. I turned to Marie.

'I love you,' I said.

She grabbed my arm with both hands and nestled her head into my shoulder.

'I love you too,' she replied.

We sat in silence holding each other until it was time to head back down the mountain, the dogs keeping us safe the whole way.

'Welcome to Kyrgyzstan, guys!' I said in my best gameshow host voice.

We were back in Osh, but this time to pick up Andrew, Alice, Paul, Connor, Bart, Irina, Alex and Ellis, the winners of a competition we'd run earlier in the trip. The prize was a five-day horse-trek through the mountains. The only issue was that none of the eight lucky winners had ever ridden a horse. 'Perfect,' I had told them all before heading out.

'Don't worry, my friend, we will provide training,' said the very friendly guy who owned the horses when I went to see him a couple of days before everyone arrived. In reality, this 'training' consisted of everyone being issued a horse on the side of a busy road, being told that 'left is left, right is right and back together is stop', and then being pointed up an enormous mountain. What followed was five days of laughter, excitement and adventure as we trekked high into the mountains, skinny-dipped in rivers, ate incredible meat and vegetable stews and pilaffs, and stayed with the nomadic families in their yurts.

On the first morning, after breakfast, having been roped

Truck It!

in along with everyone else by Paul to help celebrate his mate Connor's birthday, I stood up.

'Okay, gang, we'll be heading out in ten minutes or so, so time for us all to put our cowboy fancy dress gear on I asked you to bring.'

Of course, when Connor came back in his perfect cowboy outfit, complete with leather cowboy boots and a leather hat, we were all just wearing exactly the same clothes as before.

'Bastards,' Connor said, laughing.

The only problem was, he actually looked great.

'Well, this has backfired, hasn't it?' I said to Paul. 'He looks the absolute part.'

Even the addition of a glitter 'birthday bitch' sash couldn't ruin it.

Being able to share this life-changing experience of riding all day, up into the mountains, to come up over the ridgeline to the views down over China in the east, Tajikistan in the south and Kyrgyzstan to the north, was mind-blowing. Some of them had never been camping, or been in a sleeping bag before. So to watch them as they experienced a whole new way of living was extremely moving. Not one of us, however, could get our heads around *kumis*, the fermented horse milk drink that was a delicacy both here and in Kazakhstan. It made you tipsy if you drank enough of it, but it tasted like off cheese.

At the highest point of our trip, 3,500 metres, and with temperatures hovering around freezing, the skies opened and freezing rain drenched us all. The group made the joint decision not to split into separate female and male yurts to sleep at this camp, in hopes of keeping the ambient temperature a little more tolerable. As this group of nomads had their own dog and Red and Rubia couldn't come in with us all, we made a shelter out of metal sheeting and rocks just outside the compound. As we put the last stone in to seal in the warmth, Rubia was giving us the full-beam puppy eyes, wanting to be allowed in the yurt. But we stayed strong. We got into our sleeping bags on the hard floor, still wet and freezing, and tried to sleep.

Four hours later, we were woken by loud barks and Red and Rubia clawing at the door to the yurt. 'Your turn,' yawned Marie. In the torrential freezing rain and pitch black, I had to lead them back to the shelter and brick them back in, which made me feel extremely guilty, as they both began to shiver. The next morning, they looked at us with the biggest, saddest eyes you've ever seen. So we made sure that night, 5,000ft lower back down in the valley, and with temperatures massively warmer, we all went and slept on hammocks in the open air, with the dogs as close to us as they could get. It felt odd it wasn't just me and Marie, but it was truly humbling to see how much everyone got out of this experience.

The social media aspect of our lives often became a curse and a weight we didn't want, sometimes driving a wedge between Marie and me. But to be able to give those eight the chance to do something they would never have had the chance to do was fantastic and something I will cherish for a long time. It made all those hours of editing and crafting content worthwhile.

After five days, we drove the group back to the airport and waved them off, then headed back into the mountains for

Truck It!

one final night before we crossed to Tajikistan. And that's when the guy with the horse turned up.

'Beautiful, isn't it?' said Marie, patting its neck and in between its eyes.

'Shouldn't we tie it to the truck or something?' I asked.

'No, he's hobbled it, look,' she said, gesturing to where the rope had been twisted around its legs. 'This is the tradition here. The horses are used to it. It stops them wandering off.'

'Okay, fair enough,' I said, bowing to Marie's years of experience with horses.

An hour later, as we readied for bed and made sure we had passports and documents to hand in anticipation of an early start and a busy day, I opened the door to check on our guest.

'Ah,' I called out. 'He's literally just here.' Hoppy was munching at the grass around the steps into the truck. We hadn't checked on him for an hour or two, so it was reassuring to find him so close.

'See, I told you,' said Marie from behind her book in bed.

'Goodnight, mate,' I shouted, shutting the door, switching the lights off and jumping into bed.

'Marie! Hoppy's gone!' I shouted at eight the next morning, before she had even opened her eyes. I ran one way, then the other. Then I thought I should probably put some trousers on.

I knew how important a horse was to these nomadic people. The thought of him turning up to find we'd lost his horse was awful, however, Marie told me he wouldn't have gotten far. In a stroke of genius, I broke out the drone and set about scanning the area from half a mile above our heads. I checked in every direction across several small valleys. Nothing. We threw down the last of the coffee and I apprehensively strode ahead of Marie and the dogs as we went in search of a hopping horse among a herd a short way down the valley from us.

'I still can't see him,' I shouted to Marie, who was checking the far side of the herd.

'Me neither,' she said, throwing her hands up just in case I couldn't hear.

A field full of horses, but none of them was hopping.

'Maybe his rope came off?' I said. 'How are we going to recognize him?'

'Look for a horse with a white sock on his rear right leg!' Marie shouted.

Ten minutes later, after inspecting the rear right leg of the entire herd, we met up empty-handed.

'He must have come and got him already,' I said. Let's head in the direction he did and see if we spot him.'

So we drove off down the dusty untamed mountain tracks, winding our way down a small valley, following a river.

'Bobby, there!' shouted Marie.

'Nah, it's too big,' I replied, stopping close by to inspect one of the three horses that were drinking in the water. 'Nah, false alarm, plus it's well too far for a horse to hop. He would have had to come up the steep far side of the mountain, down this track and across the river,' I laughed. Marie agreed and we slowly set off.

Two hours later and Marie pointed. 'Bobby, there! It's

Truck It!

hopping,' said Marie, even more shocked. I screwed my face up to focus in on him, stopping in the middle of the single track. 'Surely it can't be. He's so far away.'

The horse took two hops forward. 'Oh shit!' I let out, opening the door to go and investigate.

I hopped the river and approached the horse who was head down in a field full of the most luscious grass you've ever seen in your life, absolutely stuffing his face. There was the rope looped around his ankles. There was the white sock.

'How the bloody hell have you hopped here?!' I said as he studiously ignored me. 'Marie, it's him! No way – we're over ten kilometres away!'

'What do we do?' I said as I walked back to the truck.

Marie watched him having the time of his life.

'Leave him,' she said confidently. 'If he managed to hop all the way here, he'll be fine getting home.'

As August changed to September, it was time to say goodbye to the Kaz and Kyrg Stans and say hello to Tajiki. With doubt looming in my mind, I dropped the handbrake and we set off towards the border.

'Can you imagine how fast he must be when he isn't hopping?'

And suddenly we were both laughing loudly enough that Red stirred in his bed, checking what was so funny.

'I'd definitely not have any testicles left if I rode Hoppy,' I concluded, which set Marie off weeping with laughter again.

18

Mars Landing, Tajikistan

'You, go through. You, stay.'

I stood staring at the rotund gentleman in front of me, who seemed to be suggesting that Marie was free to exit the Kyrgyzstan mountain border post into the no man's land before Tajikistan began, but that the truck and I couldn't. I politely but perhaps slightly sarcastically pointed out that we were 13,000ft up a mountain pass, with winds of -10, at dusk, and that the only thing she'd be doing if she went through the border on her own was dying of hypothermia. The green pastures of Kyrgyzstan had started to fade away as we drove up and into the harsh arid terrain we had been warned of that awaited us in Tajikistan.

His reply, as it had often been, was to shut his little window on us. This was around hour fours into an intensely frustrating

Truck It!

process in which they were adamant we had outstayed our sixty-day visa, despite us pointing out that we had seven days left. Things weren't helped by the fact we'd flown home in the middle of things. But Marie and I kept counting the days on the calendar from when we'd been stamped in to today and they kept shaking their head. We had to leave, visit the embassy, pay a fine and obtain an exit visa. He just kept waving his hand in my face with this arrogant dismissal of everything we said. I had even tried subtly waving money at him and he hadn't budged.

'I genuinely don't know what to do,' I said to Marie, with my head in my hands, looking at her now stamped passport. Luckily, after another hour of pestering, old hand-waver went off shift. And was replaced by a man who filled the entire room with the smell of cigarettes. As I went through the rigmarole of pointing at the calendar all over again, I saw him do the maths and realize we were right. Another hour and reluctant calls to their bosses later, and we were through to the no man's land that we'd have to cross to get to the border of Tajikistan.

We bounced up and up into the stark mountains, stopping at military checkpoints, each one less and less equipped, while the soldiers wore more and more layers and became skinnier and younger as the altitude increased. We passed over a mountain pass with a blizzard shooting snow horizontally across our headlights. Leaving the pass, we came round the corner, to see there was a barrier across the track.

'No way,' I said, turning to Marie, confused. 'This can't be it? Can you check the map? It looks like an abandoned military training camp, not a border post.'

Bobby Bolton

The apparent border checkpoint now in front of us appeared completely derelict – wooden and concrete huts, the fuselage of a helicopter that looked like it had been there for decades, and no lights or signs of life. We hadn't had a chance to get our horn working after it had fallen off during some off-roading in Kyrgyzstan, but I flashed the search and rescue lights a few times before hanging out of the door and whistling a bit.

A few moments later, a head poked out from the nearest shack whose door was attached only with the top two hinges. The head disappeared for a good few minutes before football stadium-style lights were activated, lighting up the heavy snow which had started to fall, and eight figures emerged. They were pretty scary-looking blokes. All of them wore black balaclavas, mismatching military jackets and had machine guns swung across their chests. I tentatively lowered myself down out of the truck, squinting into the spotlights.

'Come,' said one of the men, beckoning as he opened the gate, just as one more guy appeared with two guard dogs in a frenzy to get off the leash. I climbed back up into the cab, tentatively shuffled the truck inside the camp, and before following the senior guy into the hut, I made sure to activate one of the anti-theft devices.

As the rest of them stood still and silent, I followed the boss-man into the hut, while two of the others stayed behind us. We were in what was clearly a changing room, with boots strewn across the floor, jackets hung on bent nails in the door, and a gas blow heater turned up to full whack. It smelt of unwashed bodies and damp cold-weather gear. In the

Truck It!

corner was a broken plywood bench that had been propped up with a tree branch.

The guy took a seat behind the desk, grabbed a book from a stack and blew and wiped the dust off it. All I kept thinking was I had no idea where we were, or how Marie was, surrounded by all those guys back outside. No one knew we were here. Anything could happen. Were we even supposed to be here?

'Passport,' he barked, lifting up his balaclava to reveal a weathered face with huge bags under his eyes.

I handed over our passports and he began writing down our details. Once finished, he fussed under another pile of spare hats and gloves and found more pieces of paper before pulling out a stamp, fiddling with a few rollers and pressing his stamp on an ink pad so dry he had to hold the desk with his other hand to get any colour off it.

'Okay. Now customs,' he said, rising and pulling back down his balaclava, not quite believing that this was an actual international border and we were in the right place.

He marched me back outside into the freezing darkness, followed closely by two soldiers, before pointing to a dimly lit building at the far end of the compound.

'Okay, thank you,' I said, slightly bowing to all the soldiers.

'Jesus Christ,' I said to a very unnerved Marie, who sat stroking Rubia. 'That was a bit full on.'

As I started the engine, the floodlights were switched off and we were plunged into darkness. I weaved my way through the debris of what looked like a zombie apocalypse until we arrived at a slightly more well-maintained building marked 'customs'.

Bobby Bolton

A guy not wearing cold-weather gear appeared at the window and beckoned us in.

'Welcome to Tajikistan,' he said as I burst through the door, eager to get out of the biting wind. *Some welcome*, I thought. But at least he didn't have a machine gun. I paid a hefty entry fee, signed a few forms and shook hands before making my way back out to the truck.

'Alright, well, that was strange, but we're all good, we're free,' I said, pulling the door to as gusts of snow followed me in. About 500 metres on, we saw a flat piece of dirt and decided we'd better call it a day and drive in the daylight.

I've heard people say a place is like another planet before, but Tajikistan really is.

As we drove out the next day, Marie and I kept just looking at each other. There was literally nothing before us but vast valleys of red-tinged soil and rocks, mountains and hills in the distance. I kept expecting a little Mars lander to roll by, or to pass a US flag fluttering in the middle of a distant valley to mark a landing site.

We eventually passed a military base, presumably home to the border guards, and as we approached, a young soldier ran out to block the road, struggling to keep his AK47 under control as he did so, revealing ill-fitting baggy trousers and oversized jacket. He stood in front of the truck, holding his hand up, his machine gun hanging loosely off his arm.

I wound down the window and he spoke in Tajik, then what sounded like Russian, before giving up and radioing back inside.

'What's going on?' said Marie. I shrugged a response: *no*

Truck It!

idea. Maybe we'd forgotten to fill out all the paperwork, or this was some other sort of checkpoint?

A couple of younger soldiers appeared out of the half-opened solid metal camp gates, and then a few moments later an older guy smoking a cigarette appeared.

'Yes, hello, English?' said one of the younger guys.

'English, yes. Is there a problem?'

'No no, no problem. My commander needs you to take him to the next town. Maybe two hours away,' he said.

I half laughed, trying not to insult the guy, and turned to Marie, who was scowling.

'I'm, umm, I'm sorry we have no spare seats,' I said.

He turned to the commander of the base, who had lit another cigarette and translated the response.

'It is necessary you take him. Very important military business,' he said, making sure I understood this wasn't a request.

I turned back to Marie. 'I don't think we've got a choice here. Would you . . .'

'I'll get in the back,' she said, snatching a radio with an annoyed look painted across her face.

I beckoned the guy up.

The army commander was probably only slightly older than me and stank of booze and stale cigarette smoke as he climbed up and sat down. We set off across the surface of another planet while he stared at all the flags, maps and foreign money pinned to the truck's cab roof.

Ten minutes later, we broke into small talk, which was more like sign language. The odd English word here and there, matched with vigorous hand gestures. I learnt (I think) that he controlled 10,000 square miles of border area, though it could have been 100,000. He told me he had been shot, pulling his trousers down to reveal a nasty-looking scar on his quad.

'Tough bastard,' I said, which he nodded at, clearly not having a clue what I was saying.

I explained that I was a builder by showing him photos of things I'd built. Without asking, he took my phone and began silently flicking through all my photo albums, stopping every now and then to show me one of the dogs on a paddleboard and smile. He must have gone through every one of the 30,000 photos on there, just flicking and beaming. *At least it prevents the small talk*, I thought.

'You okay, Baguette?' I called back to Marie.

'Are we almost there? It's so bumpy in the back I'm feeling sick,' came the reply.

I was trying to drive as quickly as I could, which meant we'd hit a few potholes at nearly 50mph, sending her flying.

Twenty minutes later, we bounced our way into a little village situated on the side of a vast lake. The houses were built from mud with flat roofs. I had never seen anything like it.

'Turn,' he said, pointing, looking up from my phone.

We weaved our way through narrow alleys as locals came out to gawp at us.

'Stop,' he said, passing my phone back and finishing with 'Good', which made me laugh.

'You can come out now, Harry Potter,' I joked as a queasy-looking Marie sheepishly stumbled out of the back.

'Where are we?' she asked.

'Not sure.' As we watched, our hitchhiker was greeted by

Truck It!

a woman who stepped out of a gate and handed him a baby. 'I think we've given him a lift home,' I laughed. We waved him goodbye and drove off.

Thankfully, Marie had downloaded a load of offline maps, as we hadn't had signal since we'd entered the country. Marie studied them now, trying to work out where we were.

'I think there's an observatory in this next valley if you fancy taking a look,' she said as I aggressively fought the truck around more deep Martian potholes. The roads were concrete, which hadn't been maintained for years, presumably since the country had achieved independence from the Soviet Union in the early nineties. In places, often for miles, the locals had given up with the road altogether and formed a new dirt track alongside it to avoid the huge craters that had formed. There was clearly not a lot going on as we drove past the odd settlement of mud houses and abandoned buildings collapsing into the mud. We were still at about 4,000 metres above sea level and the altitude was giving us both a headache and that tipsy feeling, but we carried on until we turned off the highway and into the most extraordinary place I have ever driven.

Before us was a vast shallow lake and, where the water had disappeared, it had left islands bursting up out of the dirt. It was completely flat, with mountains and rock formations lifting into the bright blue sky. There were no trees, no bushes or wildlife – just the endless soil and rocks and scree. It was arid, freezing cold, and the air felt sharp and thin in your lungs. It was beautiful, but terrifying too. The altitude was also impacting the engine, as there was less oxygen for it to burn. It was grumbling as we passed an abandoned bulldozer and came stuttering to a halt alongside the observatory. The wind almost ripped the doors off as we hopped down. Red took one listen to the hurricane winds outside and refused to get out.

'That's China!' I shouted over the wind, pointing at the snow-capped mountains in the far distance.

It was incredibly impressive, but both of us couldn't imagine spending any amount of time there, like the old Soviet soldiers must have done. We felt so exposed; the wind and sun were relentless. These must have been brutal living conditions. We set off across the plateau in search of some prehistoric cave paintings and a place to park. It was so strange to feel so remote from humanity, standing and looking at marks made more than 5,000 years ago.

We were thinking a lot about time, as, suddenly, we seemed to be running out of it. Our original plan had been to take a route from Tajikistan, south through India and cross into south-east Asia via Myanmar. It was becoming clear, however, that Myanmar's closed borders weren't a temporary thing. The ongoing civil war didn't appear to be letting up any time soon. When we'd last discussed it in Kyrgyzstan, we'd decided we could either just turn up at the border saying we wanted to come in and see what happened, or we needed a plan B.

We found such a plan in the form of a 15-day transit with a guide through China from Nepal to Laos. It ran once a month and escorted a small handful of lunatic overlanders. The problem was that the weather got so bad in Tibet throughout winter that the last tour of the year was November, which had seemed so far away when we'd been planning things in Istanbul in early April. But our incredible time in

Truck It!

Turkey, Georgia and the Stans had taken us to September, and there was a real 'back to school' feeling in the air. If we missed the last tour of the year, then it shut down until the spring, sometimes as late as May.

'We *have* to make that November crossing,' I said to Marie. There's no way we'd get a visa to drive around in Nepal or India for six months, so we'd have to take a totally different route, doubling back thousands of miles, or try to arrange to ship from India to Australia, which would be insanely expensive and difficult. So, we had about six weeks to travel more than 3,000 miles across some of the most difficult terrain you can face. The time for lazing around with the dogs, climbing, paddleboarding and riding horses was over. We needed to put our foot down and drive long, hard days. Luckily, Tajikistan didn't lend itself to lazing around. We drove relentlessly for days on end, squinting in spite of our sunglasses at mile after mile of stark, sprawling terrain broken only by checkpoints.

At one, just before we would cross the border into the thin strip of land that extends up to China in the north and Pakistan on the east, known as the Wakhan corridor, two skinny Tajikistani soldiers looked the truck over, stopping to fiddle with the winch and speak into their walkie-talkies, before coming round to the front window.

'Fuel,' one said.

I opened the door and cautiously climbed down. Fuel? What did he mean? Did we have a leak?

We barely had enough to make it to the capital, which was the next place we expected to be able to fill up. Fuel stations just weren't a thing in this part of the world. Locals trade petrol and diesel out of homemade barrels and, in some cases, buckets. Mindful of what happened last time we'd bought crap fuel and bunged up the pump, and not fancying breaking down out here, I was trying to stretch our fuel reserves as far as humanly possible.

'Fuel,' he repeated, pointing at his chest.

'What?' I let out in disbelief.

I couldn't actually believe we were being asked for a bribe of fuel and not money!

'Fuel,' he said for the third time, raising his voice. This could get difficult. I just held my hands up like there was nothing I could do. The soldier frowned and turned away. There was then an awkward fifteen minutes of them on their walkie-talkies, pacing around the truck, as I sat on a wall and kept an eye on them. There was no paperwork or anything that suggested we'd be moving soon.

'Food,' he then said, again catching me off guard. I realized that we were so remote that money was of no use. This is what they needed: fuel and food. We'd tried to stock up in Kyrgyzstan with as much as possible, which was lucky, as shops in Tajikistan were whatever was for sale out of a cardboard box in front of a house. We could probably spare some if it came to it, but not much. I walked to the back of the truck and, as they peered in through the door, began to get out a couple of onions and some peppers. Then I had a brainwave. I shut the door and got back up into the cab.

'Are they asking for money?' asked Marie.

I shook my head. 'They want food.'

We both looked at these two underfed young lads. I reached under the seats and grabbed the bags of sweets we'd bought

Truck It!

to give to kids, got two big handfuls out and took them to the guards. Their faces lit up, and suddenly I wondered if they were even as old as early twenties. Two minutes later, they'd filled in the paperwork and waved us through, still beaming.

Both of us, however, were deep in thought. Here we were, so worried about how we'd complete the trip of a lifetime, and there were those two lads, underfed, in the middle of nowhere. We were so lucky, and needed to keep that in mind at all times.

'Bobby,' shouted Marie, pointing. 'It's Afghanistan!'

We had come around the corner and there, in the dirty windscreen, was the Wakhan river that marks the border between Tajikistan and Afghanistan. In the distance were huge mountains that we worked out had to be Pakistan, peering over the beautiful landscape I never knew Afghanistan had. As we bounced our way down and turned onto the river road, I thought about crossing those mountains. We'd faced some biggies so far, but these were something else.

Across the river, we started seeing Afghanis – the men in long robes and headdresses, with huge beards; the women in veils, moving quickly through alleyways. On our side of the river, men and women worked together in the fields, wearing jeans and T-shirts. It was a reminder that we were about to cross into a very different place. Elation soon turned into concern and apprehension as we both got caught up with thoughts of what might be to come.

I looked over at Marie as we bounced around on the rutted tracks.

'You okay?' I asked.

Bobby Bolton

We had spoken often about our route through this part of the world, and people had repeatedly told us that we were taking unnecessary risk by going through Afghanistan. Our conversations had always concluded with 'We'll be alright', but now, as we laid eyes on the world that lay across the river, it all felt just a little bit more real.

We had bought a full-length dress and a headscarf to cover Marie's hair to make sure we were to be respectful and attempt to blend in as much as we could. A few days before, though, she'd had a conversation with her parents, who'd told her they were really worried. It had planted a seed of doubt in Marie's mind.

'Yes, I want to go,' she insisted, smiling, but I could see it was slightly forced. 'I've been looking forward to it. I'll be fine.'

Our conversation was then suddenly cut short with an audible *'Pshhhhhhhhh'* sound coming from outside, just as one of our tyre pressure alarms started going bananas. *Ah, bugger.* I pulled over, climbed down and quickly located a small hole in the side wall of a tyre. *Damn it.*

'Is it bad?' Marie asked, leaning out of the window. We had been driving for eight hours a day for the past eight days, along roads that needed maximum concentration to avoid driving off a cliff or into a hole. The thought of dealing with this now filled me with dread. Tomorrow, after a hot meal and a sleep, things would seem a lot better.

'It's not ideal, but let's reinflate it and keep going.' So, stopping two more times to reinflate the tyre, we drove on to the capital city of Dushanbe.

We found an awkwardly small side street to park in for

Truck It!

the night, but before going in search of some good food to recharge the energy levels, I propped the rear axle with the truck's jack and blew the tyre up as high as I dared, hoping it wouldn't fully deflate overnight.

'That's tomorrow's problem now,' I announced. 'I reckon if the weight of the truck isn't forcing air out of the tyre all night, it'll be still inflated tomorrow and we can just drive and go find somewhere to get it fixed.'

The next morning, much to Marie's amusement and my complete despair, we were faced with an entirely deflated tyre, which was now so flat it had come off the bead. When Marie had come back from the tactical dog walk she'd gone on to let me calm down, she delicately suggested getting the spare tyre down. This would normally have been a great suggestion, but we weren't in the right location with the right equipment to get the 150-kilogram tyres on and off. We just had to deal with this flat tyre on our own. Somehow.

For the next two hours, I tried everything to get the tyre back inflated, but it was useless. I sat there miserably as Marie fed me chocolate biscuits in an attempt to cheer me up. I went in search of some Wi-Fi to call my dad, who after careful consideration told me, 'You can explode it back on, but for god's sake be careful.'

So, after watching a couple of videos of Russian farmers doing it on their old muddy tractors, I went back and told Marie the plan. Ten minutes later, while she and the dogs were standing a safe distance away, I sprayed a big blast of deodorant around the tyre, then lit it. *Boom!* A flash of fire and a bang. But there was our tyre, back on.

The only problem was that now our small hole had ripped

open wider into a proper hole. Me and the tyre were both completely deflated. But, unwilling to be defeated, I got to work. I took the wheel apart, cleaned the area around the hole, then, using a bicycle repair kit, glued a piece of bike inner tube to the hole with multiple patches.

'Bobby, this is never going to work,' Marie laughed as she held a phone in my face to record the stupidity of the moment. 'This is a truck. That's made for a bike, and you aren't even using it right.'

'This is literally our last option, Marie.'

One cup of coffee and a few biscuits later, I checked if it was dry and began putting the tyre back onto the rim and building it back up.

'Alright, start praying,' I said to Marie as she once again held the dogs.

BANG.

And the tyre was exploded back on to the rim for a second time.

We both held our breath to listen for any signs of leaking air.

'No way,' I said, grabbing the airline. 'No way, no way, that's worked.'

Silent, as if trying not to tempt fate, I carried on inflating the tyre until it reached our normal running pressure.

'Holy shit, that's actually worked.' I turned to Marie, beaming with pride and feeling amazing.

'Come on, James Bond, let's get out of here before you jinx us,' she said, still laughing.

'I reckon this will get us to Australia,' I said as we were barrelling along past tyre shops on the outskirts of the city,

Truck It!

too proud and too optimistic to call in to get it properly patched.

'Don't jinx us!' shouted Marie. Then, rather inevitably, only a few miles later, we heard the sound of more impending drama coming from the tyre as we hurtled along the main road.

Pshhhhhhhhhh . . .

Marie looked at me.

'Don't say it,' I said, speeding up as the tyre pressure began dropping faster, and faster.

'Now what, Bobby? It's almost flat!?'

'There!'

In a moment of pure luck, I spotted a car garage on the side of the road.

Ignoring the sign with a cross through a truck, again, I mounted the kerb and swung around in front of the tyre bay for cars as the pressure gauge hit zero. We quite literally had twenty seconds to spare. A little bit of persuasion and £6 later, and we had a repaired wheel, two spare patches and some glue.

That night, only a few miles from the border with Afghanistan, we lay and watched tracer rounds fizz through the air and listened to the crack of automatic weapons coming from over the crest of a nearby hill.

I reached over and squeezed Marie's hand in the dark.

19

The Long Road to Kabul

The explosion came low from the side of me and I dropped down into a squat involuntarily. The Taliban soldiers raised their AK47s to their shoulders and aimed at a cloud of dust coming from the truck, which had been making its way through the military checkpoint.

As my body flooded with adrenaline, I looked up to see that our escort, Mr Azizi, who was almost certainly Taliban secret police, was still leaning on the side of his number-plate-less car in front of us, calmly rolling his cigarette, not a fleck of tobacco disturbed.

Maybe a route through Afghanistan hadn't been our best idea.

Just over twenty-four hours before, we had crossed the 'friendship' bridge over the Panj river and entered

Truck It!

Afghanistan. It was the middle of September, warm, with clear blue skies above us. But we were nervous. No amount of reading blogs or articles, or talking to other people who have been, can prepare you for that first moment when you find yourself driving over an empty bridge, approaching a gang of guys carrying machine guns and standing beside a former American Humvee, now adorned with the new Taliban flag. Marie had her headscarf on and a dress that covered every inch of skin, but I could tell from her eyes how stressed she was.

We were waved over and gestured to stop by a couple of guys.

'Okay, here we go,' I said, giving her hand a quick squeeze and turning on my big stupid tourist smile as we got down out of the truck. It was thirty-nine degrees and I'd decided to wear jeans and a shirt to try to look smart.

'You. Follow,' ordered a soldier with authority. We set off in pursuit of him as he marched across a sandy area which had the feel of an old air base, flanked by crumbling buildings and surrounded by high barbed-wire fences and watchtowers. On a piece of waste ground, some stray dogs were fighting over a scrap of rubbish.

Twenty or so men were gathered by the fence and watched us as we passed, which, for the first time on the trip, made us feel extremely uneasy.

I'd seen footage of soldiers in Afghanistan and heard the term 'compound' before, but this was the first time I'd ever stepped inside one. We passed through an alleyway lined by high mud walls that surrounded the single-storey mud buildings. We took our shoes off and in our socks walked down a corridor, with me clutching a folder full of our documents, silently praying we hadn't made a terminally bad decision.

'Passport,' demanded one of the guys, who took them into the next room as Marie and I were gestured to sit in mismatched fake leather chairs.

Marie and I sat in silence while one guy typed noisily away at an ancient computer that looked like a microwave in the corner of the room, every now and then catching each other's eye.

'Come,' the same guy beckoned twenty awkward, silent minutes later.

We rose and followed him through a pair of blue wooden double doors into another room.

There, sat on comfortable chairs around a long, battered table, were six men in traditional dress. They were barefoot and the table was littered with half-drunk cups of tea. They all stared at us as we came in. My eye was drawn to the guy at the head of the table. I've faced some tough blokes on the rugby field, who revel in hurting people, but this guy truly scared me. He was bigger and older than the other guys, with a huge neat black beard and dark-set eyes. He looked very calmly at us, but I could feel my heart start to beat faster. This guy was not to be messed with.

Marie was ushered to a chair off to one side in the corner of the room. I was sat at the table. No one said anything to me. In fact, they began chatting among themselves, not even looking at me. I tried to catch someone's eye, but got nothing. If this was a technique to make me nervous, it was a good one. Time kept passing and it felt more and more ridiculous that no one had said anything to either of us.

Truck It!

'Where you go?' said one of them suddenly. I reached for the piece of paper, an itinerary from a guide called Ali, who I'd been in touch with a couple of months previously. We'd never actually finalized our plans, but I'd printed out this itinerary and the letter of invitation I'd asked them to write, hoping I could use it in the event of a situation like this.

'It's here. We have guide,' I said confidently, starting to doubt if blagging the Taliban was a good move.

He studied it for a moment, then handed it round to the others to read, before taking it back. Then he picked up his phone and began typing into a translation app, having evidently reached the end of his English vocabulary.

Are you Muslim? Is this your wife? Why have you come to Afghanistan? Are you in the army? Have you ever been to Afghanistan before?

I replied haltingly. At one point, I showed them the screensaver of my phone, which was a photo from Max's wedding of us stood together outside a church, and Marie held up her hand to show them the Istanbul ring. I felt sweat running down my back, knowing our 'fake' marriage and wedding photo would probably get us in a spot of bother.

They chatted together for another ten minutes. He lifted his phone and took the letter of invitation and started typing in the number on the letterhead. My heart sank.

'I call?'

'Okay,' I nodded. *Well, that's it,* I thought. *My bluff has been called.*

It rang for thirty seconds before he gave up, then tried twice more before he turned to me: 'Fake number,' he said accusingly.

'No, no. Busy man,' I said, trying to remain calm as the back of my knees began to sweat against the sofa.

The phone rang. I really hoped it was Ali and he had the ability to blag.

Whoever it was, he spoke to them briefly before he put the phone down.

'Okay, go bank, pay visa and road tax, then come,' he said, five minutes later, gesturing.

Thank you, Ali!

'Go, quick. Taxi outside of gate.'

We were marched outside and through the main gate where a group of locals, who were sitting around and drinking tea, stopped what they were doing and stared at us like we were aliens. Marie followed behind me, looking really uneasy.

Our escort waved towards the only vehicle and we got into a beat-up Prius with a caved-in windscreen and one welded-shut door. We drove in silence to a single-storey building, which looked like it had been a school at one point, but was scarred with bullet holes. After we'd taken our shoes off and gone in, a guy appeared from behind a curtain, grabbed our paperwork and the dollar bills before beginning to talk animatedly with a couple more guys.

Money and forms were passed quickly between the group, and at one point someone asked, 'Two people?'

I nodded back.

'Next room.'

As I struggled to put my boots back on, I realized why everyone wore flip-flops. This happened twice more. Fifteen stressful minutes later, our taxi driver came to find us, clearly getting impatient. I pointed him in the direction of where

Truck It!

I'd last seen our paperwork and dollar bills get taken and a few minutes later he reappeared waving a piece of paper.

'Come,' he beckoned.

Back at the border-office-cum-interrogation-centre, we filled out a visa form and the man with the computer declared after some slow, vigorous typing, 'Okay, done.'

We were then escorted to the truck and waved off. There was no time to debrief or plan our next move as we drove cautiously through town, past buildings peppered with bullet holes. I was very aware that the sun was starting to go down. Men appeared from one of the buildings with machine guns slung across their chests and I watched them carefully in the mirror as we passed them, making sure no barrels suddenly got lifted in our direction.

Soon we had left the town behind entirely and found ourselves approaching the edge of a desert. This was not good. As the sun got lower and lower, there was nowhere to shelter, nowhere to hide, just featureless desert with god knows what in it.

'Screw it,' I said, turning the wheel and heading off down a track, straight into the desert. I aimed for an electricity pylon but veered off at the last minute when I saw a tent at its base. In the distance through the hazy dusk, I saw a mud wall sticking out from the featureless terrain, which I guessed was used to shelter livestock. It was a metre shorter than the truck and only about ten metres long, but it was the best we could do. Darkness was fast approaching and we were desperate to find some cover to hide behind on our first night wild camping in Afghanistan.

We ate in the darkness, trying not to make too much noise,

or shine too much light. Just as we were getting ready for an early night, both exhausted from the stress of the day, Marie hissed, 'Bobby, there's a light coming.'

Oh, bugger. From out of the darkness of the rolling sand dunes, a lone torch was ominously approaching us. What or who was carrying it, I couldn't see. My heart sank in terror.

'Right, you stay here and hold the dogs,' I said as I grabbed my head torch and started walking directly to the light.

I called out *'As-salāmu alaykum'*, except I'm a northern bloke with no gift for languages, so who knows what I actually shouted into the dark. No response. I tried again. The light went out and my heart stopped in fright. I turned my head torch off, took three paces to the side and crouched down. What was going to happen next was anyone's guess. Silence. Just the sound of my own heartbeat beating quickly in my ears. The light had gone out less than twenty metres in front of me. Was a gun being aimed in my direction? Was it an innocent, inquisitive shepherd? Looking back towards the truck, I could just about make out Marie's feet on the truck steps. I walked quickly back before anything else happened.

'Everything okay?' whispered Marie.

'All good,' I said, a lot more confidently than I felt. 'Must have been a shepherd looking for a lost goat or something.'

We tied the dogs to sleep under the truck and keep watch. I made sure the big knife was at the top of the drawer, but knew it would be pretty useless against a machine gun.

We woke quickly and got back on the road the next day. We'd heard rumours of people who'd crossed the country

Truck It!

without incident, but a few months earlier a pair of cyclists had been shot dead and another pair of tourists had been killed at a popular tourist site, so relaxed we were not.

We had been told to report to a town about two hours away for some sort of permit. I had watched so many documentaries about the war in Afghanistan that it was surreal to be here. As we drove through the reddish sand and rocks, we passed through villages of squat, square mud huts. Children stopped playing, and the men would stare at us until we passed out of view. We were both so tense we hardly spoke. I was gripping the steering wheel so tight my knuckles were white.

We arrived at the town, parked the truck and walked into a government building. I was sweating immediately in my shirt and jeans. I could only imagine how hot Marie must have been. Inside, a helpful young guy gave us a long, complicated set of instructions for where to get a permit to travel to Kabul. He wrote them down in Arabic and handed me the paper. As we walked back to the truck, I saw what looked like a clothes shop.

'I need to stand out less,' I said. 'I feel like these jeans paint a target on my back.'

So, while Marie stayed in the truck, I ran in and, with a mixture of sign language and broken English, managed to convey that I wanted a traditional outfit. They measured me and told me to return in three hours.

Twenty minutes later, after driving lost around a busy town, drawing far too much attention in a big blue military-looking truck, we finally gave up and asked for directions from a group of Taliban soldiers, who were remarkably helpful once

I told them I wasn't American. It wasn't long before we finally arrived at the right building, nestled on the edge of a well-kept residential area. The homes were single-storey white buildings arranged in a compound with big gates, while the streets were wide dirt tracks, with kids running around, chasing goats with sticks or trying to launch homemade kites.

We were greeted by an armed guard, who took us to an office to an older, smartly presented guy sat in the middle of a well-decorated office.

'Hello and welcome to Afghanistan,' he said. 'We welcome you as our guests to our beautiful country. Tea?' For twenty minutes we chatted as he asked us lots of questions in fluent English. At the end of the conversation, he walked to the printer, grabbed a piece of paper, signed and stamped it, and then brought it to us.

'You are our guest in our country. Please show this at any checkpoint. It will see you pass through untroubled,' he smiled.

'Thank you. We are really looking forward to visiting. We have heard many wonderful things,' I said, shaking hands.

Marie and I both did a courteous little bow before leaving.

'Well, I wasn't expecting that,' said Marie.

It wasn't until this moment that I realized how little time we had spent together not under some sort of observation, but even here I didn't feel comfortable hugging her or holding her hand.

'How you holding up?' I asked.

'I'm alright. It's just so strange,' she said. 'We haven't seen any women and everywhere we go, they don't look at me, never mind speak to me,' she said.

Truck It!

It was strange enough for me to see, so I couldn't imagine how much stranger it was to feel it.

We decided to wait it out around the area until it was time to head off to collect the clothes I'd ordered, so we let the dogs out and gave them some water before slowly walking our way along a couple of streets, nice and slow, to give the dogs something to sniff at.

Kids came to say hello, then laughed and ran off scared as the dogs trotted up to say hello back. Rubia found it fun, but Red definitely gave off the sense that he was too old for this nonsense and would rather be in his bed snoozing.

The group of kids attracted older boys, who brought men out of their compounds, who in turn came to greet us and offer us bottles of water.

'How much do I owe you?' I said.

'No, no, this is my gift to you, brother. Please enjoy our country. God be with you,' one English-speaking father said as we shook hands and made our way back to the truck. I started to wonder whether maybe the reputation this country had among travellers was wrong?

An hour later, back at the tailor's shop, a crowd gathered as soon as we pulled up, including a food vendor, who brought us two bags of spiced French fries and two drinks: 'My gift to you!'

The group of onlookers soon turned into a crowd, and then a mob as the presence of foreigners in a big truck whipped up excitement. Kids started to fiddle with the truck and I had to raise my voice to say no as a couple attempted to open the doors and peel off the stickers we had collected. A carpenter who had been watching from the other side of the street strolled over and barked something at the kids that made them disperse. As they ran away, one of the kids called something out that made the others laugh, miming a gun shooting at us as he ran away.

In the tailor's, the suit was ready and fit perfectly. I couldn't believe they'd made a full traditional, tailored outfit in less than three hours. 'No,' insisted the tailor when I tried to pay. 'This is a gift from Afghanistan. Please. You are our guest.' And no matter how much I protested, he wouldn't accept my money.

Leaving the shop ready to hit the road in my new outfit, which suited the beard I had deliberately been growing, Marie whistled as I climbed up into the truck in my new clothes.

We set off towards the meeting point we had agreed with Ali, where his nephew and driver would meet us to accompany us on the next stage of our journey. Marie and I discussed how strange it was for there to be such kindness and generosity everywhere we looked, and yet still, we had barely seen any women.

This was heightened by the fact that we had to regularly halt our conversation as we pulled up to the many checkpoints, where guards with machine guns and hand grenades strung across their chests either completely ignored Marie, or stared fiercely at her.

After a while, she just stared out of the window as we drove past houses with bullet holes in the walls. A couple of hours later, we pulled into a dilapidated petrol station and got a nod of acceptance from a couple of guys to park over in the corner. It was well run-down, full of overgrown bushes,

Truck It!

a derelict building and a stray dog that didn't shut up, but we slept well that night with the air con buzzing away, allowing us to keep the windows shut.

The next morning, we had only been on the road about half an hour when a number-plate-less Prius flashed its lights at us to pull over. Out of the car got a young, short, well-dressed guy with delicate, handsome features. He introduced himself as Omar. This was the nephew of Ali, who had saved us at the border. He pointed back at the tall, bearded guy wearing a maroon and gold robe, who had deep dark eyes and stood by the driver's door.

'This is Mr Azizi.'

Mr Azizi bowed slightly, lighting a cigarette he had quickly rolled as Omar said hello and looked out, uninterested, into the distance. I made a mental note that Mr Azizi was not someone to double-cross. He was as mysterious as he was intimidating.

Our guides had arrived.

We were taken for lunch at a local restaurant, which was well overdue. We were almost out of food and dared not stop to buy supplies from the side of the road. We sat behind drawn curtains, sitting on cushions, and dived into platters of meat as Omar explained the next few days.

'The bad news is that the main road to Kabul is shut for trucks, so in ten kilometres, we must take the diversion. But that is past the Buddhas of Bamiyan and Band-e-Amir National Park, so it will be good.'

Mr Azizi muttered something to Omar with a mouth full of meat and juices running down his beard.

'Mr Azizi says it is maybe two hundred kilometres to

Bamiyan, but the road may be quite bad. He used to drive a truck for a living before working for the Americans. Now he works for his friend and my uncle as a driver and guide,' Omar said.

'The road is very bad to Kabul, even the main road. Last night we set off at eleven and Mr Azizi drove through the night. Drivers in Afghanistan are crazy. All they need is cigarettes and energy drinks and they can drive for ever.' Mr Azizi muttered something else. 'Mr Azizi's record is four days straight with no sleep,' Omar laughed.

It was a stark difference to my dad's world, of driving with tachographs, time-recorded rest stops and regular governmental inspections. Here, as long as you didn't kill anyone, it was fair game.

After lunch and having passed through several military checkpoints, which was made much easier by our guides doing the talking, we soon turned off the main road onto a track made up of the finest dust I have ever seen. When I went for a walk later on, and picked a handful up, it was like icing sugar. When you drove on it, you lifted a huge plume of it behind you like smoke, twenty metres into the sky. It settled on everything and everyone we drove past.

This was the main route to and from Kabul for trucks, so it was completely thronged with heavily modified former European trucks from Mercedes Benz, all driving in a single file in one direction. We stopped to look at one of the trucks they used. It had been modified to carry upwards of forty tonnes, when out of the factory in Germany it had been built for sixteen! It was like something out of *Scrapheap Challenge*, and I wanted one.

Truck It!

We quickly caught up to a convoy of trucks lifting dust high into the sky and in the poor visibility just had to drive behind them, creeping along at three miles an hour. From time to time we would pass abandoned trucks with snapped axles hanging off or exploded tyres. Sometimes the convoy would stop while some problem, hidden in the smoke ahead, was resolved. The colours were intense – the blue of the sky and the red-grey dust. The track followed a small muddy river where children played and animals drank, and we caught glimpses of women fully covered washing clothes in their compounds, while men worked the land. At slow parts of the track, there were energy drinks and crisps for sale in front of wooden shacks.

Each time the queue came to a halt, drivers would jump out, light a cigarette and form little huddles to chat. The drivers from twenty trucks ahead and twenty behind would walk in our direction and squat down to gossip about our truck.

Mr Azizi would join a group chatting and explain who were where and what we were doing, then Omar would come to chat with us and translate.

'Londonton, we tell them,' Omar laughed. 'The drivers are not very educated, so have never heard of England before, but they think London is a country, so Mr Azizi is saying you are from Londonton,' which had us all giggling.

The drivers were covered in dust and sweat, and came to ask us questions via Omar. They wanted to know what life was like where I was from and I asked them what life was like for them. They all seemed happy, with a good sense of communal camaraderie, but it was a brutal life living on the bread line in a country still grappling to settle down after decades of conflict.

Hours and hours went by, and pit stop after pit stop continued, so we got to know the nearest ten drivers quite well.

'Do you want to come and chat?' I turned to ask a rather depleted-looking Marie at one of the unplanned convoy stops. She just shook her head and stared blankly out of the window. I could tell she was exhausted from being ignored. It made her feel like a ghost.

As the sun started to lower in the sky, I flew the drone and saw one continuous line of trucks behind us, stretching back for miles and miles, heaving around the harsh dry terrain.

Day turned to night as we continued to bounce our way along difficult mountain tracks, past villages and fields, and the trucks began to turn on their lights. Blue lights, green lights, purple lights, red lights, some flashing, some spinning, some strobing – they lit up off every corner, each side of the trucks. It was like an incredible lightshow, better than any trip to Blackpool illuminations.

I told Marie something one of the drivers had said, and she replied, 'This is the only country so far where I feel like you are just having a totally different experience to me.'

I couldn't do anything about it. The way women were treated felt foreign and insulting, but in their culture was the norm. Nevertheless, I couldn't stop the rising feeling of guilt as Marie went back to stroking Rubia in silence.

It was early evening when we were stopped on a narrow stretch of track, while some of the drivers were eating a meal of bread and onions, when we heard the distant scream of

Truck It!

a siren I'd only ever heard on the TV. At once, everyone got up and sprinted for their vehicles.

'Go, quick!' said Omar and we ran back to the truck.

We anxiously watched as trucks began to leap out of the way as two pickup trucks came hurtling down the dirt track towards us in a huge dust cloud. Each one had two massive Taliban flags mounted on their bonnets and a chunky rear-mounted machine gun. Blue and red flashing lights aggressively lit the dusty night's sky as men on the rear waved vigorously at the truckers to get out of the way. I desperately started the truck and held the accelerator to get enough pressure for the handbrake to release, but as they came towards us I realized I wasn't going to be able to move in time. The first pickup truck bounced down our side, but the second truck came to a stop directly alongside us.

I looked to my left, across Marie sitting in the passenger seat, and found myself eye to eye with a Taliban soldier holding a fifty-calibre machine gun. He wasn't wearing traditional dress, but a black balaclava, boots and combat gear – also as many grenades and as much ammunition as it was possible to strap to himself.

I watched his eyes narrow as he scanned the inside of the truck.

Time stopped. I didn't breathe, not knowing who or what was going to move next.

He slowly turned to Marie, looked directly into her eyes, and said, '*Salam alaykum.*' His voice was deep, slow and menacing, and sent shivers down my spine.

'PSHHHTT.'

The noise came from the truck to signify the pressure had reached its limit. I dropped the handbrake and lurched forward to make space for them to pass.

Neither of us said anything, but we were utterly shaken.

The unpredictability of what was going to happen next in each situation was almost impossible to judge.

That night, Omar told us that Mr Azizi wanted to cook a traditional meal for us. We had pulled over on a wider section of the track, just outside a little village where twenty or so trucks changed tyres, cleaned air filters and welded repairs. As the welding and grinders threw sparks into the air, we went and bought meat, tomatoes and bread, always with the locals hurrying to do what Mr Azizi said. Then when we returned to the truck, he climbed into the back and set about cooking a feast.

As we waited for dinner, Omar turned to me, smiling: 'Do you know why we are being treated so well?'

'No, how come?' I said.

'Because he looks like the Taliban FBI,' he laughed back.

'The Taliban FBI?'

'The Taliban have these spies who don't carry any weapon on their shoulders to blend in, but they are the most devout and religious members. They deal with anyone who is not following to the law or keeping their religious belief. The Taliban originally came from the mountains; they are usually skinny men with crazy looks in their eyes, just like Mr Azizi.'

That night, after we had eaten and were back in the truck, I turned to Marie.

'The Taliban FBI?! What the hell are we doing, Marie?!'

The next morning, we set out again and, at one point, we

Truck It!

were ambling through a village when we realized that our guides had become separated from us somewhere back in the convoy. It was a hot day, and Marie had lifted her headscarf a little. At that moment, a guy with a huge, unkempt beard came walking by at the side of the road. I saw him notice Marie as he walked past. The next minute he jumped on the side of the truck, hanging onto the wing mirror, staring into the cab. I stopped the truck in shock, which almost threw him to the ground.

He shouted at me angrily, gesturing at Marie, as I held my hands up and said, 'Londonton, Londonton. Tourist.' But he kept looking at me with his crazy intense stare. I noticed that he had a notebook and a pen in his top pocket and a metal knuckleduster hanging off his hip. I held one finger up and retrieved the radio from the cab and tried to hail Omar, but all I got was static. The guy was still ranting and I had no idea what we were going to do. This guy was about to lose the plot.

'Hello, Bobby?' Omar's voice crackled, finally.

I explained that we had been stopped by this intense guy in a village. Omar told me to give him the radio. Omar barked something to him and suddenly his face turned from a deep scowl to a beaming smile. I laughed at the sudden change, it was so comical.

When Omar and Mr Azizi arrived, they shook hands with him, had a little joke, laughed and waved goodbye.

'Omar, what the hell was that?!'

'Taliban FBI,' laughed Omar. But Marie didn't laugh as she lifted her headscarf back up to cover herself.

At one of the checkpoints, we got out to stretch our legs.

I was still shaky from the last one after I'd shouted at a group of guards trying to force their way into the back of the truck, almost braking the handle in the process.

We were only a couple of miles from the end of the track, watching them search trucks for members of ISIS, when there was an explosion. The only reaction from Mr Azizi was a calm glance in the direction of the blast. Following his gaze, I saw that one of the trailers that had driven past us had an exploded tyre. I laughed in relief as Mr Azizi winked in my direction and carried on smoking, completely unfazed.

I went to change my underwear before we moved off again.

We spent that evening in Bamiyan, and the next day walking round the infamous Buddhas, the sixth-century statues that had been destroyed by the Taliban in 2001 but which were now set to be restored. It was an incredible location, but, as so often, we felt so conflicted by what we saw. In the afternoon, we decided to cancel our trip to the Band-e-Amir National Park after Omar told us women weren't allowed to bathe in the beautiful blue water. It was a tiny thing in the scheme of things, but the gap between how Marie and I were treated was just so huge. We decided instead to go straight to Kabul, where Ali, the guide, owned a hostel opposite the Iranian Embassy. After a dash across Tajikistan and a week of stressful driving through rural Afghanistan, we were well overdue a break.

At one of the final checkpoints, we were caught off guard when the commander invited us to have tea with him and his officer. After checking my 'wife' could come, we agreed. The commander was an infinitely calm guy in his late forties,

Truck It!

who smiled frequently. A carpet was brought out of nowhere and laid down in the shade under a tree next to the road, just as the soldier reappeared without his combat uniform on, revealing a beautiful black traditional outfit with fine embroidery.

As Omar translated in a low rumble, he told us that the commander and the other officer had been best friends since they were children and had joined the Taliban at the same time. He spoke of how much they were looking forward to the future and to peace. He explained that they fight men who came in war, but welcome me who came in peace, like a brother. When he heard that we had cancelled our plans to swim, he offered to send us an escort so that Marie could swim, which we politely declined.

'No matter what religion, our god has filled our heart with peace and with his guidance we shall continue to bring peace and keep our country safe,' he said.

'We would welcome you to join our army if you would like? You seem strong-willed and we would teach you well. We would give you a house and treat you as our own brother. Would you consider it?' Omar translated to me and raised his eyebrows.

I laughed in surprise but didn't want to appear disrespectful. I said that, many times, outsiders had tried to invade Afghanistan, and they had all failed. So, if I was going to be taught to fight by anyone, I would want it to be them. As Omar translated, they smiled, nodding. 'Maybe in another life, but in this life, it is not the path I am on. Thank you, but no,' I said, still trying to register if I had just been asked to join the Taliban or if I was in fact dreaming.

Both men nodded in agreement and topped our teas up.

I asked one final thing: 'If you had one message for people in my country, what would it be?'

Both men looked at each other momentarily after Omar had translated it, before the main guy came back almost immediately.

'We do not need to force a message upon you. Go from here and see what you can of our country, meet our brothers and our sisters, visit our beautiful places, and form your own opinions and share *that* message. I already know what message that will be.'

I couldn't believe it. The confidence that guy had in his country was incredible. I certainly wouldn't have been that confident giving the same message in England. I would have said, 'Don't go here, avoid there . . .'

We drove on to Kabul and the hostel. Being behind twenty-foot-high walls, secured by big metal gates and a 24/7 armed guard, brought an enormous sense of relaxation. For the first time in days, possibly weeks, it was as if we could fully relax. Marie took her headscarf off and walked around the room, stretching out. We talked about how crazy the past couple of days had been and how on edge we had both been constantly. It felt incredible to be able to be intimate with each other, to hug or to touch each other's hands without worrying who was watching us. That night, we slept a deep, uninterrupted sleep.

20

Dinner with the Taliban

'Where are you from?!'
 'Why are you here?!'
 'Is this your wife?!'
 'Are you a spy?!'
 The questions were relentless.
 We were surrounded by thirty or more Taliban soldiers with guns as we sat on a rickety old bench blinking in the bright floodlights. Surreally, there was a volleyball court in the field next to us. I tried to answer but immediately there was another question fired from a silhouette looming over us. To my side was Marie, in her headscarf, which made it hard to exchange looks in the way we normally would when faced with trouble. I sat slightly forward on the bench, both hands on one leg, and looked back up at the crowd with my

head held high in an attempt to give the impression that I wasn't panicking as I answered: 'England. Travelling. Yes. No.'

One guy, who had especially wild eyes lined with thick black kohl, kept twisting his head to the side like a dog every time I answered in a way that sent shivers down my spine. At one point, he came striding over and put his foot on the bench, leaning down to peer at me. I tried to telepathically send Marie the message that she should look away, absolutely sure he was going to go at me with a knife. In what was becoming a regular experience in Afghanistan, I wondered if this might really be it.

The day before, we had decided to take the dogs for a wander around Kabul, which was not a sentence Marie or I had ever thought we'd utter. We spent the morning eating delicious food and drinking gallons of tea. Omar came along too to help translate and explain some of the history of this fascinating city. I was immediately surprised by the groups of women that were walking around unchaperoned. From talking to others who had been to Afghanistan, this was illegal even in the city, and in the rural areas we had been in so far, that certainly seemed to be true. But we were served by a woman at a smoothie place, and I could tell Marie immediately felt slightly more at ease. We strolled past amazing smells coming from the wood-burning grills of the bustling restaurants that lined the streets, and I saw hardly any buildings with bullet holes here, the rubble that we had seen frequently in rural areas was much less apparent, too. We stopped at a shop to replace our horn, getting one that was originally designed for a train, then headed back for more food and tea. That night, we went out to a restaurant where the owner sat cross-legged in the front window, butchering the meat for that night's meal on a wooden tree stump between his legs. There we ate a traditional meat dish, using bread instead of cutlery and plates. It was delicious and I went back to the hostel covered in food and incredibly full.

The next morning, after a breakfast of bread and yoghurt, it was time to leave, and the first thing we needed to do was get a permit to allow us to drive to the border with Pakistan. Omar guided us as we wound our way through a maze of streets of central Kabul towards the government building we had to go to. The closer we got to the centre, the higher the blockades became, the more barbed wire was tangled above us and the meaner the soldiers looked. We were searched multiple times, Marie noting how the women were especially thorough.

'Ah, another fondling,' she said as we were searched for a third and final time.

Finally we stepped into a lush green courtyard with men going about their business, calmly walking with pieces of paper from building to building. It was so different to the intimidation of outside. We went to three different buildings with Omar until finally, in a small office, a neat, well-spoken man came in and told us that 'the Head of Affairs' would like to meet us. We both rose to our feet and I brushed my beard into shape and fussed with my hair as we walked into the lion's den, an office five times the size of the one we'd just been in.

Both walls were lined with leather armchairs and there

was a huge desk at the end. A big guy with a huge beard sat to the side of his desk, again looking very causal, stroking his beard with one foot tucked underneath him on the seat. He asked us through a translator how our journey had been. I gave him a very heavily edited version of our trip so far, telling him how delightful his country was and how everyone we had met was excited for the future. He nodded in a way that suggested I'd said the right thing.

A couple of minutes later and we were heading back out through the maze, clutching our precious piece of paper. We were hoping this meant we could travel out of the city unaccompanied, but when I went to say goodbye to Omar and pay them, he told us they would be accompanying us to the outskirts of the city in a way that was very much not a question. We didn't want to make things difficult for them, so we hopped into the truck and headed into the chaotic morning traffic of Kabul. No traffic lights were working, and police were focused on security not traffic control, so it felt a little bit like giant bumper cars as vehicles and trucks wove around each other, often on the wrong side of the road.

Eventually we got to one of the main exits out of the city, a roundabout followed by a main road. About fifty metres out, I clocked that there was a height restriction barrier up ahead. I honked the horn to get Omar and Mr Azizi's attention but by the time they noticed, we were only a few cars from the barrier. Mr Azizi got out, lit a cigarette and then disappeared into a hut. He reappeared two minutes later, waved Omar into the car, did a tight three-point turn and we heard the radio crackle to life.

Truck It!

'Follow us,' said Omar nervously.

'No way. He's joking, right?' said Marie as Omar craned his neck out of the window as their car started to pick its way back up the side of three lanes of traffic coming in the opposite direction.

'Oh, Jesus,' I said, doing my own three- (seven-) point turn to get the truck around, laughing at how ridiculous this was.

Twenty metres or so back up the road, with their car paused waiting for us, a couple of soldiers appeared from the central reservation, opened a gate and helped stop traffic as the Prius and our truck dashed through.

Slowly it dawned on us what was happening. As we laughed and gasped, it transpired that Mr Azizi had spotted there was no height barrier on the traffic coming the other way on that busy city centre road. So, we found ourselves driving directly into three lanes of oncoming traffic as it parted around the car in front of us. At one point, a few guys with guns slung on their shoulders appeared in a pickup truck and went to talk to Mr Azizi, but came away as if it was an absolutely normal thing. I had hoped that getting our piece of paper would mean we could blend into the background. Instead, as cars beeped, hundreds of staring eyes watched us from the cars that came by.

When it was time to get off the road, we drove the wrong way up another street before bumping over the central reservation and forcing our way into the traffic on the other side of the height barrier. Just outside of the city, we pulled over and said our goodbyes and profusely thanked Omar and Mr Azizi, who nodded, while leaning against the car and smoking.

Bobby Bolton

We were heading east by around 200 miles via Jalalabad, which was then only about fifty miles from the border with Pakistan. The plan was to find somewhere to stay there and then cross tomorrow morning. The liberalism of Kabul soon felt like a distant memory and we were back to being stared at suspiciously by everyone we passed. Every time a jeep of men with machine guns went by, I'd grasp the emergency hammer we'd moved to within an arm's reach of my seat. Marie was totally silent, staring straight ahead, trying not to give anyone anything to object to. We didn't see anywhere around Jalalabad where we could park up, so we kept on going in hope of somewhere quiet to hide for the night. Easier said than done in Afghanistan in a ten-tonne big blue truck.

As dusk approached, however, about ten miles out from the Pakistan border, I spotted a track that led off into some hills to our left. We turned off, hoping there would be some sort of natural cover where we could park up and get some sleep before our border crossing the next day.

Five minutes turned into ten, which turned into fifteen, and then into twenty. Alarm bells started sounding louder and louder as we headed into what felt like proper badlands. It was just a single dirt track leading through single-storey buildings until even those thinned out as they became abandoned. It just felt like the sort of place where you'd come around the corner and find some nasty men with guns. As we got to the top of the hill, we saw three middle-aged guys dressed with skullcaps and waistcoats stood next to a small pickup, taking pictures of the beautiful sunset over the vast open valley in front of us. They were the only people we'd seen since leaving the highway.

Truck It!

'Let's just wait here until they go, so no one spots us going down that way.'

'Good idea,' Marie agreed.

I pulled up ten metres away from them. 'I'm going to get out and take some pictures to not make it feel weird,' I said, getting out.

I walked up to the side of the track and stood looking at the impressive view in front of us. The guys who were chatting and laughing among themselves looked over a couple of times, before I caught their eye and smiled and waved back.

They began heading over, so I walked towards them to greet them and break the ice.

We all said hello, even though only about three English words were said, one of which was 'Londonton'.

They were all interested in the truck, so I waved them over, thinking the quicker I give them a quick tour, the quicker they would be on their way, as the light was fading fast.

They oohed and aahed over the truck. I grabbed the globe from Marie and gave them the full 'We started here in France, drive to here now, and finish over here.'

They were all giddy, like kids – taking photos of the truck and us and the globe. They said they were all from Pakistan but couldn't return.

I showed them a couple of videos I had taken of the truck, on the drone, which spurred one of them to lift his phone out.

What he showed me I wasn't expecting. It was, without question or doubt, a terrorist group's propaganda video, full of soldiers stood in a line saluting, with clips of them running around shooting machine guns, and even one of a rocket launcher shooting at a target. At a couple of points he pointed at a guy in a balaclava, then to himself, then a few clips later to one of the other guys stood watching the video.

'Facebook friends?' the main guy said, which made me laugh.

'Yeah, sure,' I responded, chuckling and looking at Marie, who looked extremely worried.

He gave me his WhatsApp number, which came up with his name followed by the letters 'TTP', which I recognized from the video he'd just shown me. A quick google later on revealed this guy was a member of the Tehrik-i-Taliban Pakistan, which is an umbrella organization of various Islamist armed militant groups operating along the Afghan–Pakistan border, where we now found ourselves. The friendliest of the terrorists slipped his phone into his pocket, took two steps back from the circle that had formed, looked around, before pulling out a handgun and turning towards me, still smiling.

Time froze as I tried to work out what my options were. Run? No good. Jump under the truck? Possibly. Grab one of the other guys stood next to me and disarm him? *Oh, come on, Bobby, this isn't a James Bond film.* Only a couple of seconds passed, during which time I decided that my strategy would be 'stand completely still, smiling maniacally'. He slipped the magazine out of the bottom and cocked it. I tensed every muscle in my body. Then he flipped it around and held it, handle first, out to me.

'You want to shoot?'

I'd never felt relief like it.

Truck It!

'Yes,' I squeaked. 'Yes, sure thing.' I glanced over to the truck, where Marie was almost certainly watching and assuming I was about to be shot. He handed me the weapon, pointed my arm in the direction of a mud bank and flicked off the safety. Him and his mate pulled their phones out to record.

The gun leapt in my hand as I fired it.

'Cool,' I said, turning back to him with the weapon lowered.

'Again!' he said, excited, as he put one more round in the chamber, released the magazine so I couldn't empty the rest of the bullets in his direction, before I turned around and fired again.

I handed the pistol back to him, still shaking with relief and adrenaline and fear. They started watching their recordings, comparing and laughing. Then one of them shouted as a white truck was spotted in the distance.

'Goodbye, Londonton,' they called, after shaking my hand vigorously and sprinting off to their truck.

I did the same.

'Bobby, I can't believe you,' said a noticeably distressed Marie, fighting to hold back tears. 'What the hell were you thinking? What if he had pulled the gun on you and shot you?'

I just nodded and climbed up into the truck. 'I'll explain later,' I said, getting ready to start the engine.

But, at that moment, the white truck came to a stop alongside us and I swung around to see four heavily armed guys staring back at me.

You have got to be kidding me, I thought.

The biggest guy, who was unarmed, dressed in all white

239

in the passenger seat and clearly the boss, muttered something. Three of the doors burst open and the four of them got out and approached us. The guy in white slowly opened his door and took a few slow steps towards us, staring at me the whole way. One of the men must have been a bodyguard, because for every step the big guy took, he followed three steps behind, one to the side, keeping two hands on his weapon at all times.

'What are you doing here?' he said in English.

He muttered something to the other two before waiting for an answer, and they started to snoop around the truck.

'We are tourists. Looking for somewhere to camp,' I said, trying to smile.

Marie whispered something to me and handed me the permit we had got from Kabul and the original letter from day one. But it didn't work as expected. The big guy took it from his bodyguard who had come to collect it, and he raised the pieces of paper high in front of his face, so he didn't take his gaze off us for a second. He stood a few paces back and took a seat back in the open door of the car before lifting out his phone. For the next ten minutes, he made three loud phone calls. We stood completely still like statues, terrified of what was going to happen as the other soldier made a perimeter around the truck. The phone calls finally finished and there was silence for what felt like an hour, but must only have been five minutes.

Moments later, a beat-up old car came bouncing down the track and one of the armed guys flagged it down. He peered in a for a few moments and then started speaking to an occupant, who came over to us.

Truck It!

'Hello, my name is Usef. What are you doing here?' the guy said very quickly.

'Oh, thank goodness you speak Engl—'

'What are you doing here?' the guy interrupted. 'You should not be here.' He looked like a schoolteacher and was clearly very nervous. 'You should not be here,' he repeated.

'We are looking for a quiet place to camp. Tomorrow we go to Pakistan,' I replied.

He translated what I'd said to the big boss, who gave a slow, menacing nod in return.

'Who were those men you were talking to?' Usef asked.

'I don't know. They stopped to take a picture with us.'

He translated the sentences and looked suspiciously back in our direction. At that, the big boss man thumbed his phone, looking like he was texting someone, before turning to me with a 'No problem, no problem.'

I took that to mean one of two things: either there was genuinely no problem, or there was a really big problem.

Surrounded by a variety of menacing men glaring at me, it felt like it was going to be the latter of the two.

Just as the sun finally began to set, a siren began growing louder and louder as a green pickup truck erupted from around a hill, driving extremely fast with five Taliban guys inside, one on a rooftop-mounted machine gun and two balaclava-clad guys hanging off the back.

At that moment, I accepted my fate. I mentally started preparing myself for what was to come, as guilt began consuming me that I had brought this fate also upon an innocent Marie, and two dogs. I tried to remain calm as the pickup skidded to a stop and the big guy rose to his feet, pulling a prayer mat from the inside of the car.

Two men spread out from the pickup, seeming to help cordon off the area, three of the men approached the truck, one man went over to the big guy to receive orders, while the machine-gunner and sidekick stayed in position. We were now surrounded by twelve Taliban members with guns and one schoolteacher who looked equally as shocked as us at what was happening.

The two main guys conferred for a moment before the schoolteacher was given something to translate before being dismissed.

'You will now follow this pickup truck to their camp. They will keep you safe there. It is not safe here for you to sleep. You must go now,' he said, and walked off, not giving me time to respond and looking equally as concerned for my safety as I felt.

The big boss had set up his prayer mat and, with his bodyguard and other soldier still stood on guard surrounding him, began to pray.

The eight guys who had come from the pickup were whistled and beckoned and all jogged back to the vehicle, jumped in and began driving back down the track from the main road.

'I'm so sorry, Marie,' I said, looking over at her. I didn't know if she was too pissed off or scared to answer, but she didn't respond for the fifteen minutes back to the main road.

With sirens blaring and blue and red lights flashing, we followed the pickup back the wrong way down a fast main

Truck It!

road as the two spare guys on the top waved excitably for traffic to get out of the way.

We turned off the main road, past a series of concrete blockades, watchtowers and checkpoints, and came to a halt in a courtyard, just outside the gates, through which we could see another, smaller, inner courtyard. I turned off the engine and turned to Marie. Her eyes were big and scared, as I'm sure mine were too. *What the hell was going to happen next?*

'Come now. Follow,' shouted the passenger from the pickup truck as we came to a halt and more soldiers appeared from inside the compound.

We quickly threw the dogs in the back, praying this wouldn't be the last time we saw them, and followed our escort through the gates as a procession of heavily armed soldiers followed us. We entered the inner courtyard, which was surrounded by high concrete walls with watchtowers and spotlights. It had a metal walkway all the way around, and sentries on guard peered down at us. Then we were led to the side of the volleyball pitch, and that's when the questions started.

I tried to keep calm and answer while meeting their eyes and eventually a few of the soldiers lost interest and the questions began to thin out. Then a senior-looking guy walked over and shouted at all the lads, most of whom then dispersed, leaving only a couple who squatted on the pitch watching us. We sat in silence for some time as they spoke hurriedly to each other.

'Big boss is coming. Wait,' called one of them.

We must have sat in silence for an hour, the only sound

the chatter of our guards swapping over. Then someone came and spoke to our guard and he nodded and came over to us.

'Big boss tomorrow,' he said. 'Come.' Then he beckoned us to follow him. We did so, expecting at any moment to be taken to a cell or an interrogation room, but instead came into the inner courtyard, where there was a bench and a table.

'Here, please eat,' he gestured. 'You are our guest.'

We sat down and two guys brought over two plates of food and a jug of water.

'What the bloody hell is going on?' I whispered to Marie as the guards disappeared. 'Is this an interrogation, or dinner and drinks?'

We both started eating, dipping the flatbreads into a lentil curry.

'Oh my god,' said Marie. 'This is delicious.'

She was right. It was some of the best food we'd had our entire trip. After half an hour, someone came and cleared the plates.

'Boss come tomorrow. Come.'

We followed another guy back out towards the truck, which I was incredibly relieved to see one more time – on this occasion drawing less of a crowd.

'Sleep,' the guy instructed, beckoning towards the truck. We didn't need telling twice.

As we opened the door, the dogs were eager to get out, but we pushed their snouts back inside.

'Sorry, dogs, you're going to have to cross your legs tonight. We have to keep our heads down.'

It was gone 10 p.m. by the time we ended up back in the

Truck It!

truck. We closed all the blinds, got into bed and stared at the ceiling.

'What is going on?' said Marie. 'Would they bother giving us dinner if they were going to interrogate us?'

'I don't have a clue. But whatever is going to happen, we can't change it. Let's try to get some sleep so we're prepared.'

She took hold of my hand.

'I love you,' I said.

'I love you too.'

And we both lay with our eyes open, imagining what was coming next.

21

A Relaxing Drive Through Pakistan

'No, no, no!'

The police officer's eyes widened as Marie screamed at him.

'That's it. You keep saying you are keeping us safe, but I have never felt so unsafe in my entire life.'

She stood with her hands on her hips with a look that anyone who has ever known a French woman will recognize as the moment things have gotten serious.

'You are going to give me our passports and we are going to leave. Now!'

Marie was not going to be messed with. Through all those hours of being stared at, ignored, and talked past and about in Afghanistan, we had been concentrating on getting to Pakistan, which in our heads had become the light at the

Truck It!

end of the tunnel. The only problem was, now we'd reached it, there was just a load more tunnel.

We had woken up in the late September sunshine in Afghanistan at six the previous morning and had sat on the steps drinking a freshly brewed cup of coffee when our escort from the night before arrived.

'Go now. Big boss not coming,' he gestured animatedly. 'You must go now.'

From the look in his eye, we knew he was serious, so we ran about drinking big gulps of scalding coffee as we threw everything into the truck. Then, after waiting far too long for the air pressure to build, we set off. We were waved through the checkpoints and soon found our way out onto the main road.

'Was that a dream?!' I grinned as we hit the open road. 'Never mind coffee, I need something much stronger.'

'I thought they were going to shoot us and bury us on that hill,' said Marie.

We drove for the border as fast as we could in hope of a break from the madness of Afghanistan.

Precisely an hour and thirty-three minutes later, we were standing in a cattle pen at the Pakistani border as a goliath of a guard grabbed a six-year-old girl, raised her to his chest, and threw her back over a six-foot wall to the crowd on the other side.

Under a low metal ceiling which was already heating up in the morning sun, we were in utter bedlam.

Marie was slumped on the floor, exhausted. I've been involved in a 15-versus-15 brawl at a rugby game, with the coaches and some of the crowd getting stuck in, but that didn't come anywhere close to what we were stuck in the middle of right now.

A lane to our left was crammed with people trying to leave Afghanistan, and a lane on our right brought people in the other direction. Every single guard was a giant, well over six foot tall with barrel chests, and about ten of them were in our immediate vicinity, slapping, punching, grabbing and throwing people around, sweating profusely in the heat. When they found a child with a satchel full of cigarettes, they were picked up and thrown back over the wall to where they had come from. Porters pushing wheelchairs were slapped if they didn't move quickly enough. Bags were grabbed and tossed, clothing ripped, and all of this was to the soundtrack of shouting, wailing and children crying.

'Hello, sir, my name is Muhammed. How are you?' said a guy as he shut the gate for the central pen behind him among the chaos. He was in his early sixties and looked like a university lecturer in his glasses. Either side of our tiny holding pen were the raucous incoming and outgoing border queues. 'Sorry for the noise,' he said politely.

I laughed in his face. I couldn't control myself. 'Don't know what you're on about. It's lovely here,' I said sarcastically, just as an elderly man was slammed against the metal fence behind where Marie was sitting. 'Nice bunch of lads,' I said, pointing towards the guards.

'We don't want the Afghan people here,' he said gravely. 'They cause a lot of problems for us. I'm so sorry, we won't be here long.' After five minutes, the sanctuary of our cattle pen among the madness was opened and he beckoned one of the guards, who blocked a route through the mass of

Truck It!

writhing, screaming people and we ducked out of the chaos through a side door. I'd be lying if I said I wasn't grateful for the special treatment, but I felt sorry for those still out there who weren't receiving it. It was utterly brutal.

'I try not to spend much time out there,' said our escort sadly.

We turned down tea and after getting a document signed that said we agreed not to sell the truck or commit tax evasion, we were led back out, across the chaos and to our truck.

'One last thing,' he said, setting off my Columbo alarm immediately. 'We want to keep you safe, so there will be an armed escort from here for thirty kilometres until you reach Peshawar.' He shut the door, smiling. 'From there, you will be released to do as you please. Good luck and welcome to Pakistan!'

He then signalled for the gate to be opened, but we only made it a couple of metres before a different guard stepped in front of us with his hand raised.

'Oh, what now?!' said Marie, very much ready to leave Afghanistan behind. A van reversed out in front of us and opened its doors. Four men got out and opened the back of the van, then lifted out a coffin and carried it back past us.

'Ah,' said Marie.

'Well, that's something you don't see every day,' I said as the deceased was carried across no man's land from Pakistan to Afghanistan.

As the final arrangements were made, we were met by a huge policeman with a comically large handlebar moustache.

'Hello there,' he greeted us. 'We are here to arrange an

escort for you to keep you safe. Are you able to take one of my men in your vehicle?' I turned to Marie, who was nodding in tired agreement.

'Okay, please bear with me five minutes. Welcome to Pakistan.' We waited for ten minutes before he came back out with a younger colleague, who handed me up a package of newspaper, which I passed over to Marie. 'This is a gift to you from Pakistan,' said handlebars.

'It's a kebab,' whispered Marie. Starving, we wolfed it down.

'This is your escort.'

Stood in front of us was a tall, skinny kid, who must have been no more than nineteen. His uniform looked like a pair of curtains on him and he had enormous feet that made it look like he was wearing flippers. He saluted, which caused his machine gun to drop off his shoulder, and he then got tangled trying to get it back in place.

As he climbed up into the truck, I whispered to Marie, 'Well, I feel safer already.'

As we navigated leaving the border, our guide pointed every now and then, but spent most of the time grinning out of the window and waving at people he knew. I was tired, and wired from so much adrenaline, and so when a truck came at me on the wrong side of the road, only swerving out of the way at the last minute, blaring his horn, I swore my head off at him and gave the two-fingered salute. I turned to our escort, who was smiling away. But then it happened again. And again.

'Baguette, can you hear me?' I radioed to her in the back.

'Yeah, what's up now?'

'Can you just check if Pakistan drives on the left?' I said.

Truck It!

'Hold on,' she said, then, after a minute, confirmed: 'Yeah, they drive on the left, why?'

'No reason,' I said, veering over to the other side of the road, our guide smiling all the time, completely unaware of my naivety.

We made good time to Peshawar, where our guide got down and waved goodbye, smiling the whole way. But then the police officer held his hand up. 'Your next escort is ready.'

And that was the exact moment that Marie's last shred of patience was exhausted.

'Hold on, we were told we were to be escorted to Peshawar and we were free after that. So what is this for?' she said, her voice loud and her eyes fierce.

'It is for your safety, miss,' he said. 'You must be escorted.'

Walking along the hard shoulder towards us was another pickup full of armed guards. Marie huffed as only the French can while the two groups said hello to each other.

'Where are you going?' repeated the new head of the next escort as the guy we'd been speaking to walked off.

'Is this a joke?!'

The police officer blinked in surprise. 'Miss, it is for your safety. We . . .'

'We told your boss: We. Do. Not. Want. An. Escort,' her feathers now well and truly ruffled.

'Miss, it is—' he started to say again.

'Lahore, we go to Lahore!' I loudly interrupted, to save his life more than anything.

I had been fiddling on my phone trying to come up with a plan.

I beckoned Marie to get back in the truck before we ended up in a shouting match.

'What did you say that for?' she hissed angrily.

'Lahore is on the other side of the country – it's like twelve, fourteen hours' drive away. No way they're going to escort us that far. They'll take us a bit further and wave us off down the road.'

Marie snorted in agreement but continued to shoot daggers at the guys in front. 'I know it's hard, but let's just try to stay chilled out,' I said.

Five hours later . . .

'This is bloody ridiculous!' I shouted as the escort in front of us peeled off to reveal another escort taking their place. For five hours we had been kept moving, without a chance to stop, or give a second for the dogs to take a wee.

'Bugger this for a game of soldiers,' I said, and overtook the pickup full of armed guards and turned left off the highway. We were in the middle of rural Pakistan. I picked up speed round the bend and accelerated away, catching sight of a couple of pickup trucks with lights flashing, racing to catch us up.

Over to one side, I saw a cluster of half a dozen trucks pulled over on a large gravel area, clearly parked for the night, and pulled in to join them.

'This'll do. I just need a break,' I said as I pulled over, the pickup trucks following us in. 'Marie, just let the dogs out for a quick wee, then jump in the back with them and shut the door behind you. I'll tell them we are stopping here.' As I jumped down, the pickups came screeching to a stop next to me, men with machine guns jumping out, covering me in

Truck It!

dust. I stood upright, hands on my chest, squinting my eyes as the dust cloud was lit up with flashing blue and red lights like fireworks.

'Sir! What are you doing? It is not safe. It is very dangerous.'

'Not safe?! The only thing not safe is you,' I shouted, pointing at the soldiers holding guns. 'Tell them to point that away from me and take their fingers off the bloody triggers!'

Two young soldiers were dressed like eight-year-old boys playing army in their nan's back garden.

I turned back to the two main guys who were on the radio, taking another deep breath to calm myself.

'Sir, we are tired,' I reasoned. 'We just want to sleep. Please understand. There is no law against us sleeping here, nor are there laws that we must be escorted. Please leave us. We will continue on our own tomorrow. Thank you.' I bowed my head politely in their direction, turned to lock the truck and walked round to get in the back.

'Sir, sir, it is not safe, you must come with us, sir, sir,' I heard before I jumped in the back, shut and then locked the door.

Marie was sitting on the floor cuddling Rubia, holding back tears.

'Why won't they leave us alone?' she said, exhausted. 'I'm just so tired.' I held her as she shook with tears. 'I just feel so sorry for the dogs.' We both stayed that way until there was a loud banging on the back door.

'Sir?! We must go. Now!'

Then another, deeper voice. 'Sir, I am the chief of police. I am afraid you cannot stay here. It is not safe. I cannot permit it.' I took a deep breath and went to unlock the door.

Bobby Bolton

Outside was a guy in his early fifties with a balding head and a well-kept beard who held himself like he'd been in some tasty situations. I shook his hand firmly and looked him in the eye.

'Sir, I understand you are here for our safety, and I am grateful. But I want to be left alone, so what do I need to do to make that happen?' I said, calmy but firmly.

'You cannot stay here I'm afraid. It is not safe.' I blinked twice, about to lose faith. 'If you come with me, there is a hotel you can stay at. We will leave you there, it is safe, and tomorrow you can leave undisturbed and travel at your will.'

I raised one eyebrow. We had been passed like pass-the-parcel since we'd arrived in the country.

'I give you my word,' he said. 'Please. Follow me.' Then he turned and shouted orders at the rest of his pissed-off-looking men.

Two hours later, I had tried to repair the damaged bathroom door and had cleaned the toilet, though I couldn't do anything about the mysteriously stained bed sheets and we were just about to go to sleep. I had also realized why we were having such a problem. All of the research I'd done about Pakistan had been on places in the north of the country I wanted to visit. But what I'd realized was that all of the blogs and website articles were written by people who had flown in. The reason we hadn't encountered any horror stories about driving up through Pakistan was that no one ever seemed to bloody do it. We had been concentrating so much on Afghanistan, we'd taken our eye off the ball for Pakistan. And now we were paying the price.

Truck It!

I was standing in my boxer shorts when there was a knock on the door.

I opened the door to an unarmed guy, wearing a smart uniform, surrounded by three armed guys. 'Hello, sir, I am the chief of police. We are here for your safety.'

'Ha! Of course you are,' I scoffed back, having heard the same line two hours earlier.

'We are here for your safety. I am here to insist these men guard you on shift all night. You must pay for their room to stay.'

Despair turned to anger. 'Listen, mate, we were hanging out with the Taliban last night and shot a gun with a group of terrorists who you are now trying to protect me from. I definitely do not have to pay for their room.'

'Sir, you do not have an option. They will stay here all night taking turns to guard you. If you do not pay for their room, they will sleep on the floor.'

Damn it. He had called my bluff, as I definitely didn't want that. I looked into the corridor where two young lads stood. This wasn't their fault. 'And tomorrow?'

'Tomorrow, sir, you are free to go,' he said.

The next morning, after a night of no sleep, as our escorts played Candy Crush with the volume set to high, we were walking towards the truck when a guy wearing a uniform stepped out.

'Good morning, sir, we are here for your safety to escort you.'

'Oh, why don't you just f—'

Marie cut me off: 'Thank you, we will be five minutes.'

Over the next couple of hours, seven separate escorts came

and went, ranging from smartly dressed police officers to two blokes in a pickup who we weren't even certain *were* an escort.

'Can we stop for the rest of the day somewhere?' Marie asked. 'There is a camp hostel thing ten kilometres away.'

The next time our escort changed, I showed them the location of the camp and told them that was where we were heading.

'Okay, there is a bridge three kilometres up here. We will leave you there. Cross the bridge and head straight to the camp. We know there. He is a good man.'

I let Marie know the good news, and a few minutes later, we reached a wide, well-built bridge crossing the slow-moving river that flowed through the Swat valley.

'Apparently, it's the Switzerland of Pakistan,' said Marie, researching the area on her phone. Our escort kept their word and turned around, waving goodbye as we reached the bridge.

'Good lads!' I said. 'Finally.'

We turned off the main road where a little pill box with a policemen was checking and letting through cars.

'No tourist,' the guy said.

I slapped the steering wheel. 'Oh, for god's sake.'

Marie tried to negotiate, as we were minutes from our destination, but it didn't work and the guy was uninterested.

He soon started to get agitated, as we were blocking a line of local cars behind. 'Move,' he insisted.

We turned around and set off up the nearside of the river. I checked the map on my phone. 'Okay, there's a bridge up there, half a mile away. We'll just go to that one.'

Truck It!

Five minutes later, we were flagged down at a big military and police checkpoint.

'Where is your escort?' the first guy demanded.

We both let out a laugh in disbelief and didn't bother explaining. The boss was called and I handed over both passports as requested, before calmly explaining our situation.

'You must wait here. You need escort. You cannot proceed,' he said, walking off with no interest in our complaints, slipping our passports into his pocket.

'Well, we made it about a mile,' I said grimly to Marie, who had once again lost all sense of calm and looked like she was about to grapple with the next person who spoke the word 'escort'.

I was starting to feel a bit like a spoiled brat. It's not like we were paying for the escorts, after all. They must have genuinely wanted to keep us safe. But it meant we didn't have a moment to stop or even slow, to take the dogs out, to use the toilet, to meet or talk to anyone, or any of the things that had made the trip so joyous. Instead, we were rushed along, unable to do anything all day. We waited for two hours, with the guy holding our passports. And *that* was when Marie lost it.

She stormed over to the guy, shouting and snatching our passports back.

Marie jumped in, slamming the door behind her. 'Let's go,' she said.

And it was that exact moment that the gearstick went into flopping fish mode and broke.

'I think the bracket has snapped again,' I winced as I struggled to hold it in first gear.

As armed guards began to swarm around us, waving, I found first gear and we set off. We drove at 6mph back to the bridge.

'You cannot pass,' the guard reiterated.

Now completely distracted, as we couldn't drive anywhere if an escort should turn up out of thin air, I set about lifting the cab off the truck and, wearing a pair of rugby shorts and Crocs under the sweltering forty-degree midday sun, began repairing the truck once again.

'I'm going to call the embassy,' Marie shouted over to me as I had my head deep in the engine bay.

Now, I've never called the embassy, nor did I think it was going to help, but our only option was to go back the way we had come, through all the police escorts, and back to the first town after the border. I couldn't bear the thought.

'They are going to call me back in ten minutes,' Marie shouted as I was rewiring a cable which had been cut as the bracket snapped.

I finished the repair, declaring it good enough for the time being, and walked the dogs over to the river for a drink.

'Sir. Dangerous. Not safe. Go,' shouted the guy at the checkpoint.

It was early afternoon by the time a military guy arrived in an SUV with blacked-out windows and spoke to the checkpoint dude, who pointed in our direction. He walked over to us, taking off his CIA-style sunglasses.

'You can cross the bridge and go straight to the camp. Make sure the owner calls us to let us know when you have arrived,' he said, matter-of-fact, before getting back in his car and driving off.

Truck It!

'I love the French embassy,' I said as we drove off over the bridge.

We arrived at the camp, which turned out to be a peach farm nestled on the edge of a small valley just outside of town. The guy greeted us with a huge smile and a handshake.

'I am sorry to hear of your troubles,' he said. 'Welcome to my farm. You can park here, we will feed you and you can walk through the fields with your dogs. You are safe here. It is completely free, I insist.'

After the past forty-eight hours, I felt my bottom lip wobbling as he showed us to the shower room, and his son brought us tea and biscuits. I'd been on high alert for so long now, but the past two days had been the craziest of my life, and my body was feeling it.

'This means a lot, mate,' I said, shaking his hand. 'I can't tell you how much.'

For two days, we slept, ate and drank among the peaches. But then, when it was time to go, there were the escorts again. We spent a whole day driving too fast, too slow, almost crashing, shouting, arguing, apologizing and negotiating toilet and food stops. It was immediately exhausting. At one point, we were flagged down by a guard at a checkpoint, who grabbed his machine gun and approached.

Marie took her moment to jump out and use the toilet in the back. The twitchy soldier, on seeing her walk down the side of the truck and open the door, shouldered his AK47 and aimed it at her.

'What the hell?!' I screamed as I jumped in front of the barrel of his gun with my hands high above my head. 'We are tourists! What's the matter with you!' I shouted at him.

Still with the gun pointed at us, but slightly slower this time, he got on the radio. Neither he nor I moved for a minute before a few more guys burst out from a side gate.

'Sir, you can't be here. It's not safe. You need an escort,' he said.

The boss man quickly made a few 'calm down' motions with his hands and barked some orders, which got the men to stand down, and a few walked off.

'I'm sorry, you have come at a very dangerous time. You are not safe here,' he said.

'I'm sorry, mate,' I said, shaking my head. 'I don't understand what we are in danger of. Your men shooting us? No one seems to be able to explain, and the most unsafe we feel is when we are around the police.'

He ignored my question, told us to wait and called for another escort.

Two hours later, just before dusk, I'd had enough. I pulled off down a narrow track in a tight valley. We had managed to escape our most recent escort with the cunning ruse of shouting 'no thank you' and driving off.

We turned off down the track, both giddy like children that we were about to spend the first night alone, unguided or unguarded since the day before the puncture drama back in Tajikistan.

'There will do – or there. Actually, let's get a bit further away from the road,' I said as we continued down the concrete narrow track.

'Oh, bugger.'

We had come within sight of a house and compound at the bottom of this narrow, steep valley.

Truck It!

'Okay, I'll walk down and see them and see if it's okay to stay here.'

Marie nodded and shouted to be careful as I walked off down the track.

As I approached the compound, the children stopped playing and ran inside, one reappearing momentarily with an older guy. 'Hello,' I said to the man, who seemed to be in his mid-thirties and had a big smile as he greeted me in return.

'Please,' he said beckoning me inside his compound to where five other guys were lounging around drinking tea.

As they brought me a cup of tea and a cup of milk, I tried my best to mime where I was from, where we had driven from, and where we were heading, which was all received with nods and noises of agreement.

As I felt the conversation dying, I tried to explain that we wished to sleep halfway back up the valley, which they flat-out refused, insisting instead I should sleep in their spare room. I managed to negotiate bringing the truck to their yard.

Marie screwed her face up in disbelief as I arrived back at the truck on the back of a motorbike ridden by our new best mate and host. I just laughed and said, 'Just go with it . . .'

As we parked up and after Marie had said hello to the very excitable kids and the dogs were released to have a sniff around, we were invited inside again.

More small talk broke out, now with the assistance of a translation app, and Marie was invited to meet the women of the house, who were behind another gate leading to another part of the house.

Marie excitably walked off, led by our friendly host, retuning twenty minutes later with a painted hand, wearing a head scarf and a massive smile.

'They are so nice. There are so many of them, maybe six or eight. They made me feel so welcome and were all fussing over my hand-painting and headscarf which the younger girls gave me.'

I thought how long it had been since Marie had really seen a woman, never mind talked to one. I kept having to remind myself that, however I was feeling throughout this part of the journey, it was nothing compared to what it must have been like for her. This was a rare moment of calm and safety.

That evening, we ate and drank and laughed as these complete strangers opened their home to us. We waved goodnight and went to bed with our hearts full of joy. Marie had the most enormous grin, the sort I hadn't seen for days.

Early the next morning, just after dawn, we were woken by a banging on the door. I stumbled towards it, bleary-eyed, to be greeted by a very pissed-off-looking guy in an army uniform.

'Sir, what are you doing here?! It is not safe. You must leave!'

'Who is it?' called Marie from the bed as I shut the door in his face.

'Marie, you're never going to believe this . . .'

22

The Banks of the Ganges

We watched as the old woman's head covering caught alight, the flames licking higher and higher until her body was just a dark shape in the fire. Two men stayed to watch the body burn and the others turned and walked back up from the banks of the river.

We had been standing beside the Ganges, watching the wide slow water from its sandy banks when the old woman's body had arrived on a stretcher. One young guy about my age who was holding the front corner of the stretcher beckoned another man over to take his place. He stood and removed all his clothes so he was just in underwear, walked into the river and, without anyone saying anything, fully submerged himself. Wiping his face of water, he nodded and the four stretcher-bearers slowly walked into the water and then, as others built the fire, submerged her, before carrying her back and laying her onto the ready-to-burn bonfire. With no prayer, no words, no fuss, the young guy had lit a torch, walked round the pyre four times, and then lit the fire. Without thinking about it, I took Marie's hand as we watched smoke rise into the air from the six other funeral pyres, so thick it felt like it was dusk.

'This is one of the most intense things I've ever seen,' I whispered to Marie.

As we stood in silence, we saw other bodies arriving on stretchers as people stood around the fires. Some appeared to be family members, others locals. Some heavily decorated Hindu monks sat silently meditating, too, as the mid-October sky darkened.

Two weeks before, we had been woken by the police guard knocking at the truck door in Pakistan. We had dressed in silence, and then Marie had given them a very loud piece of her mind. As I packed up, I heard fragments, as did most of the valley.

'Safe?! Safe?! We were safe until a bunch of twenty-year-olds with machine guns turned up . . . Leave this wonderful family alone, now!'

When I glanced outside, the entire police guard were standing with their heads down, like schoolkids getting a dressing down from the head teacher. Yet again, I thought how lucky I'd been to be up that mountain in France at the exact moment she was.

After a while, I went out and put my hands on her shoulders.

'Come on,' I said. 'Time to go.'

Truck It!

She was so angry she was close to tears. 'It was so nice, the girls with their heads uncovered, they were laughing. I haven't heard women laughing for days. And then they turn up with guns.'

'I know,' I said, hugging her.

The family came out to say goodbye, so I went and told the police guy we'd meet him at the top of the road in five minutes. Then Marie came out of the truck with two necklaces and put them around the girls' necks. She hugged them, whispered something to them, before finally waving goodbye as they disappeared back into their compound.

For the majority of our time in Pakistan it was the same story of escort after escort rushing us through the country, until finally, in the far north, they faded away. There, in the high mountains, we could finally breathe. But neither of us could quite forget the route to get there.

We stood, amazed, in the Katpana desert, the highest in the world, its sand carved into a knife's edge by the wind. We hiked up to Marsur Rock, a slab of stone that cantilevers out over a huge valley with a river winding through it. But even though we were 3,500 metres up, with snow-capped mountains all around us, we were both distracted, partly from what had just happened, but also from what was to come. A bomb had gone off at a nearby airport, and there were protests and riots between government and anti-government forces. Both of us had got incredibly intense food poisoning on our way north and were only just recovering. Plus, our Indian visas were looking like they were going to be a little more complicated than we had initially thought.

Most of the time, we'd been able to wing it with visas,

which was lucky, as we couldn't do much else. In Tajikistan, there'd been a bit of an issue, before eighty dollars judiciously doled out to the various border workers did the job. But to get into India via a land border, we needed to have visited an embassy for a physical sticker. As we got closer to the border, we got word that upwards of 80 per cent of applications made for land crossings were being turned down. At an internet cafe, we managed to read a few forums and speak to a few fellow travellers who in some instances were flying back to Europe to visit their home countries' embassies to secure visas, all of which was taking four weeks plus. But there was no way we could leave the dogs for that long.

'Is that it?' I asked Marie, as we both sat, stumped.

But then we heard about a 'fixer', and he explained his plan. He would look after the dogs for twenty-four hours, parked up three miles from the Pakistan border. We would take a taxi to the (recently bombed) airport and fly twelve hours west to Abu Dhabi, then on to Mumbai. There, we would get stamped in, stay for one night, then fly back, pick up the dogs and drive into India, having exploited a slightly ludicrous and definitely not very environmentally friendly loophole. So, forty-eight hours later, still full from eating far too much extremely spicy food in Mumbai and having been reunited with two very excited and confused dogs, we found ourselves at the famous Wagah border. There, every day, there is a complex ceremony as both the Pakistani and Indian army march and raise flags in a symbolic show of strength, before the border is formally opened for the day, and the same thing happens again when it is closed.

Getting into India felt like turning a new page. Perhaps

Truck It!

because it was such a relief to be able to move slowly. We stopped and visited the most incredible ornate temples as we drove through the northern Punjab. We talked to people and laughed and smiled. There was so much noise and movement and life. Pakistan had felt so skittish and intense. This felt joyous. We were also, finally, feeling properly over our lucky-dip curry food poisoning and were starving. And even as we watched the vendor washing his silver tray in gutter water, we couldn't resist the street food. We ate heavily spiced fried potato and bread, sucking air into our mouths to cool it down, and then danced in a crowd of men and women with their faces painted with the Indian flag.

We couldn't take too much time, however, as we only had four weeks to cross India and Nepal and apply for our Chinese visa, which was already sounding complicated. Our visa agent said that anyone who had spent fifteen consecutive days in either Turkey, Afghanistan or Pakistan ran the risk of their application being passed to Beijing, which would take months – and months we didn't have if we were to cross the Himalayas that year. Unfortunately, we had the hat-trick, having stayed for more than fifteen days in all three . . . For this exact reason, both Marie and I had tried to get hold of a second passport. I had managed to organize one for myself, which was pristine and without a single stamp in it, but Marie hadn't had time to do the same. We were going to have to hope that we could sort it on the Nepalese border.

It was at this point that it was beginning to dawn on us how much it was going to cost to ship the truck to Australia. We were being quoted US $15,000 from Singapore, the same from Malaysia. Even from Thailand, which was the cheapest, came in at 8,000.

'And that doesn't include docking fees, customs charges, port entry,' said Marie. 'Blah blah blah. Expect to pay an extra 4,000 dollars on top of everything else.'

I held my hands up in surrender but she kept going.

'Please note, it is extremely important to clean the vehicle sufficiently to pass customs. "No dog hair, no seed, cutting, stick, twig, dust, mud or dirt can be on the truck as it arrives at Australian customs. We've had to deal with a few horror stories where customers have had to pay an absurd amount of money to have their vehicle recleaned by a third party."'

I took a big sigh. 'That is going to be the hardest part, money aside. I've not cleaned it since I bought it.' We sat in silence, thinking about the sheer amount of multinational dust and dirt there was currently in and on the truck.

However, as we were both firm believers in crossing the bridge when you get to it, we put that to the back of our minds.

'Enough of that,' I said. 'We have a decision to make. Taj Mahal or mountains?'

Of course, we chose mountains. But first, it was time to travel through the most populated place I had ever been. As we drove past Shimla, along roads thronged with thousands of cars, bikes, tractors, trucks, cyclists and homemade contraptions I didn't know the name for, they all blew their horn every two seconds. With my driver window wound down, I had to wear ear defenders, I was genuinely worried the noise would damage my hearing. Even as we got to the mountains, it felt as if every part of the roadside was being

Truck It!

used for something. We drove for hours unable to find anywhere to park up. For us, it was astonishing, but for the locals it was just normal. And when we did find somewhere to stop, people would casually nip in the back to come and say hello, or look through the cupboards to see if we had anything interesting. All of which was done with massive smiles and no real malice.

It was like magic. One time, I pulled over into a kind of traffic stop in the middle of a motorway, feeling like there we would surely have a moment to ourselves. But we'd stopped for thirty seconds when a gang of kids appeared and started jumping on the front of the truck and laughing. This attracted some men who were walking by, who came over to talk to them, which meant some motorcyclists stopped, which meant some cars stopped. Within two minutes, we were the centre of a crowd in the middle of the motorway. We politely said our goodbyes and drove on. We were going to have to drive enormous distances if we were to make the crossing through China and into south-east Asia before winter. I reminded myself that, on our first day, we had driven pretty much the entire length of France. We went to bed that night utterly exhausted.

Wild camping at the foothills of the mountains on our way north, I woke up at about 2 a.m. with intense stomach cramps. I sat up, dizzy and nauseated. I went outside for some fresh air, tripping over Red, but only made it three metres before I fell to one knee and vomited. At the same time, my body let me know it also needed to use evacuation method number two, so I scrabbled as far into the bush as I could and squatted down. For the next few minutes I felt like I had regressed to a non-human state. I was just a big tube full of liquid emptying at both ends. It was so bad I found myself praying in the pitch darkness.

As the latest batch hit the floor, my ears turned my head back in the direction of the truck, just as the door flung open, light flicked on and Marie fell on her backside down the three steps, making sure she didn't drop the toilet roll, but once again standing on Red.

'*Putain!*' she shouted as she shuffled past me, holding her backside.

The next day, we were mostly silent, queasy and had to stop regularly to run into the bushes clutching toilet paper. I'd heard all the travel jokes about 'Delhi Belly', but my god. For the next two weeks, with only a couple of minor exceptions, we ate nothing but eggs on toast. A week in, we chanced another delicious roadside curry and were both fine. But the following night we did the same and were both sprinting into the dark early that morning. After that, we decided we couldn't risk it. We had both already lost so much weight, and we couldn't seem to find shops that sold anything other than bread, coke and nuts. We felt at risk of scurvy.

Long days, with little food and dizzy from food poisoning, all blurred into one feverish dream. I spent it wondering what I was really doing. Part of the trip was supposed to be working out what I wanted to do with my life. Marie and I had long conversations about it. Luckily neither of us aspired to live in big houses and drive fancy cars, so we agreed we just wanted to keep having experiences like this. Well, not exactly this – retching into the bushes every few hours – but seeing the world and meeting people. We were so close to

Truck It!

the finish line, but, if I was honest, a lot of the joy from the early part of the trip had been sucked out of it now by the complex processes to follow and pressure we were facing. We were afraid that we might make it all this way and then fall at the final hurdle. The idea that it would all have been a waste of time. That I should grow up, stop dragging Marie and the dogs around the world on a whim and get a proper job. Those days full of laughter in the cool mountains felt a long time ago and our time in Afghanistan had really taken it out of us.

And Marie was having similar thoughts. What was she doing, giving up the life she had planned for someone she'd bumped into up a mountain? We were both exhausted and pretty low, sitting slumped in silence as we drove down from the Spiti valley into the lowlands when we came around a corner and Marie sat up.

'Bobby, I think that's the Ganges.'

We had gone down to take a closer look. We knew that the Ganges was a holy river and people came to bathe in it. I said I wanted to dip my toes in, so I could say I'd done it, though Marie shook her head. And that's when we saw the smoke from the first fires.

We stood, held in a trance, watching the men as they carried the bodies into the water, then lifted them gently onto the pyres and lit them. It wasn't completely silent. They talked and laughed as they performed their duties. Sometimes monks in orange shawls with huge wild beards and pierced ears, their faces covered in brightly coloured paint, would come and speak. It was a constant process, as the water kept on moving, the ash from the fires mixing into the mud of the river. It was impossible not to think about the sheer number of times this exact thing had happened for hundreds of years. About how, right this moment, in every country on the planet, people were going about their lives, engaging in their rituals and traditions. That there were billions of people all thinking that the way they did things was normal. And how there was no such thing as normal.

On our way back up to the truck from watching the cremations, we were both silent. But this time it felt as if we were still processing what we had seen. We both knew that any trip of the sort we were on could only ever take in the very tiniest fraction of the places we were seeing. But coming across something so ancient and so alien to our own traditions felt like the point of the trip. I realized that's what travel does. It takes us out of the things we have become deadened to through familiarity and it reminds us of the sheer unlikelihood of any of this. It takes us apart and puts us back together in a slightly different order. There are all sorts of reasons why people can't just travel wherever and whenever they like. But I would say to anyone, if you can, if you're wondering whether or not to take that trip. Take it. It is the greatest gift you can give yourself: the gift of rediscovering the wonder of being alive.

23

Everest and Other Adventures

'No, sir, I'm afraid we can't help you.'

The border guard had a look on his face that made my heart sink. I had walked up to him, blithely smiling my best idiot tourist smile, with my pristine 'spare' passport.

'I can only stamp if there is an exit stamp from India.'

I made my smile even broader and more stupid. 'Yes, but India would only stamp next to their entry stamp, so how am I supposed to start a new passport? I am running out of space and need your help,' I lied.

'Sir, we cannot help.'

We had entered Nepal at the beginning of November, through essentially a borderless border. For the first time, crossing into a country had felt like passing through just another rural village, with perhaps a few more police hanging around than usual.

I went out to where Marie was waiting for me by the truck and shook my head.

'What now?' she asked.

'Dunno. But we've got until we get to China to think of something,' I said.

We had originally missed immigration and customs, only to be stopped a couple of kilometres down the road by checkpoint guards, who explained that we needed to look for a small building within a row of shops and restaurants. We found it, incongruously, next to a pen of Asian buffalo.

We had big plans to park up in the mountains and just decompress after the intensity of Tajikistan, Afghanistan and Pakistan. As we drove through Bardiya National Park between the border in Nepal and Pokhara, the last big city before we hit the mountains properly, I was astonished by the number of monkeys, deer and birds we saw. The park ranger had explained that we had a ticket that meant we had to make it through to the next checkpoint in eighteen minutes, so no stopping, which meant I was barrelling along, pointing at animals as Marie shouted, 'Slow down, Bobby!'

'Elephant, Marie! Look, an elephant!' I shouted, turning to look at her as the truck swerved and bounced along the terrible road and she grimaced.

At Pokhara, a vibrant scattering of buildings spread between Phewa Lake and the Annapurna Mountains, we parked the truck and almost immediately found a smoothie bar. After our food poisoning and egg-on-toast diet, the thought of some fruit and vegetables was like a dream. We wandered from shop to shop, buying bread and hummus and pasta, which we hadn't seen for months. It was very much needed. We had both lost a lot of weight, and were nothing more than muscle. We decided that the strict budget we had imposed could be broken for a couple of days as we tried to get our strength back. So, at the gateway to the Himalayas, for two days, we ate and ate and ate. Then it was time to head north to the Annapurna mountain range.

After a brief detour into the Nepalese high altitude army training base, which we managed to explain and apologize our way out of, we went for a hike in a valley that two French motorcyclists had told us about. It's one thing knowing that the Himalayas are higher than the Alps, but then you get there and there's a mountain and it just keeps going and going and going. The scale is just totally different. As we stood looking down over the valley, with the colossal wall of the mountain stretching up for thousands of metres, taking up almost the whole of our field of view, we decided we would set out early and hike up the hill for sunrise. And I knew that there was something else I had to do, too. So, as we hiked back down, Marie chatting excitedly, I was silent, distracted.

'I'm just going to check on the gear lever for an hour or so,' I lied as I lifted out my tool bag and got into the front of the cab. 'I don't want it breaking up here.'

I went through my tool bag, looking for anything suitable – trying a jubilee clip, twists of wire. Nothing was right. Then I saw the multicoloured prayer flags we had tied between the sun visors. I took my knife and began cutting small ribbons from the bottom of each flag. Then I knotted the ribbons around the keyring, pulling them as tight as possible. From time to time I bashed the hammer and turned the engine off and on, so it sounded like I was fixing the truck.

Forty-five minutes later, with both thumbs cramping, I was done.

The next day, we set our alarm for 4.30 a.m. and hiked for two hours up to the perfect spot on the side of the hill. The only problem was that thick cloud had come in overnight and blocked our view across the valley. I suggested we wait a bit and see if it cleared by sunrise.

'Let's stick a coffee on and wait,' I said. 'It's going to be beautiful.'

But half an hour later and the cloud was still there.

'I think it's a waste of time,' said Marie.

'Give it time, it will clear,' I said, offering prayers to the weather gods. But, as the light began to pour across the valley, we could hardly see the mountain dead in front of us. Then Marie poured water over the lighter, which meant no coffee. Perhaps this wasn't the moment after all. I said let's wait another half an hour. Then another. But by this point Marie was getting impatient, so I admitted defeat and started to pack up.

Then, just as we were lifting our packs to leave, the sun broke through the cloud and we saw across the valley. It was like looking down over the whole world. I had heard the expression 'take your breath away', but at that moment, I truly understood it for the first time. It was like a physical feeling of awe and wonder. The view below and back up and overhead was like something out of a Hollywood film.

'Marie, this is so magical,' I dithered as we both walked back the ten metres or so to the summit and viewpoint, with the wall of mountain erupting high above us, now out of the clouds. I knew now was the moment.

Truck It!

I slowly dropped my bag to the floor and took the coloured ring out of my pocket.

'Marie . . .' I said, holding back the tears of joy that were appearing as I got down on one knee. 'I want to share the rest of my life with you. I don't want the adventures to stop and . . .'

'What is that!' she squealed, giggling and pointing at the colourful ring which looked like it was going to be too big, even for her thumb. We both laughed at how ridiculous it was to be doing *this* with *that*.

'Well, yeah, sorry! I knew this was the place and it felt like the right time, but it caught me off guard so I had to wing it,' I said, gasping through the tears of laughter that had appeared.

'It's perfect,' Marie said as she leaned over Red, who was sitting between us, completely unaware, with a stick in his mouth.

We held a long hug, neither of us wanting it to stop.

This was just meant to be a solo trip to give me time to reset. But this journey was turning out to be life-changing. Life-saving.

Meeting Marie had altered the course of my life from the terminal implosion I had found myself in. What lay ahead of us, neither of us had the faintest of ideas, but it didn't matter. We lay in the heather, looking up into the glaciers, clinging to the side of the 23,000ft-high mountain overhead, taking in the moment.

'I can't wait to see where this goes,' I said as Marie lay on my chest in silence, lost in her own thoughts.

'Me neither,' she whispered.

Bobby Bolton

A week later, I walked into the police station in Katmandu.

'Hello, I hope you can help me. I had my passport stolen and I think I now need a new entry stamp in my new one,' I said, trying to look as innocent and stupid as possible. It turned out that my fiancée and I had come up with something.

24

Tibetter or Worse

'He says you must pay,' said the junior officer sternly. 'You crash into Chinese Army. If not pay. Go jail.'

I watched as the senior officer shouted for a good while, while panic continued to rise in us both. We were on the side of a road in Tibet, and our guide was uncontactable.

I gulped a dry, nervous gulp.

'Please tell him I'm awfully sorry,' I said, doing my best Hugh Grant impression.

It was the very end of November, and we had been winding our way along a road in Tibet, looking out for an upcoming petrol station, when the road had suddenly narrowed, and in spite of both of us pulling over as far as we could go, we'd clashed mirrors with a truck coming in the opposite direction.

'Ah, bugger,' I said as I pulled over.

Then I saw the canvas at the back of the other truck open and ten angry, shaven-headed, fit-looking guys were jumping out and marching over in our direction.

'Oh, double bugger.'

I checked my mirror and saw the wing mirror guard had been knocked off and was lying in the middle of the road. So, I jumped down out of the truck and ran out to retrieve it, where I was surrounded immediately by soldiers. Angry ones at that.

'Oh, triple bugger,' I dithered under my breath.

I picked my way through them, saying, 'excuse me', 'dreadfully sorry', 'beg your pardon', grabbed the wing mirror, then headed back towards our truck, hoping that one of them wasn't going to shoot me. Then I mimed that I was going to drive to the petrol station. It was there, on the forecourt, that the senior officer gave me a dressing down.

We had arrived in Tibet, four days before, as part of an informal convoy of those travelling overland. We bounced around on the terrible Nepalese roads for about eight hours out of Katmandu, and though they weren't the worst we'd experienced – that prize when to Afghanistan – they came a close second.

The border is at about 10,000ft above sea level, and we knew we were getting close as we encountered the end of the truck queue. A trucker's village had sprung up around the border with little huts functioning as guest houses, or offering tyre changes, cigarettes and money exchange.

Once we had been given permission to pass through, the final stretch was just a narrow mountain track until we reached a hut that resembled a Sunday league football changing room from the 1970s in desperate need of renovation. A shout, a stamp and a wave later and we were out of Nepal, heading into Tibet, which isn't recognized as an independent nation by China, but is governed as an autonomous region. As we watched the shack recede in our wing mirror, we arrived at what looked like an enormous airport terminal in the mountains; the Chinese border.

Lampposts bristled with CCTV cameras and the border guards wore immaculate uniforms, but it was time to see if our passport ruse had worked.

The one bit of drama came when I had forgotten to check my phone for pictures of Buddhist temples, which we'd been told might be looked unfavourably upon. I realized I had no idea which temples were Buddhist and which ones Hindu, so had to feverishly delete every picture of a temple I had as I queued before they demanded my phone. They then searched the truck thoroughly and we were forced to give up our magic all-purpose wooden blocks, which had got us free of mud so often.

After the closest thing to a strip search we'd experienced on the trip, the dogs were given the all clear, our passports were stamped and we suddenly found ourselves driving on pristine tarmac.

Without any major problems, we would now pop out of China fifteen days later in south-east Asia, marking the final leg of the journey.

We went to meet our Tibetan guide, Sanghe, which was mandatory if you wanted to travel overland through Tibet, and he directed us through the neat streets as people got on with their days. Marie and I talked about the fact that no one was milling about. In most other countries, there were people sat about watching, or talking. But here, everyone seemed to be on a mission.

Sanghe explained that 'autonomous' had a very different meaning here, and that life was very controlled in lots of ways. Sanghe was in his early forties and from Lhasa. He seemed to have a healthy dose of vitriol towards those who ruled his country.

'There is an old Chinese saying,' he said. 'The emperor is very powerful. But the emperor is very far away.' Then he gave a mischievous smile.

With the huge snow-capped mountains in the background, neat green meadows and spotless buildings, it reminded me of Switzerland, which I hadn't been expecting. At one point, I saw a drone buzzing above us and pointed it out to him.

'I thought drones were banned here?' I asked.

'Oh, they are,' he said. 'That's the government "taking care" of us.'

He pointed and I saw that down the street there was a police car and a blacked-out SUV with someone taking pictures of us out the back. Maybe we weren't in Switzerland after all.

The plan was to head along the Myanmar border, then south-east towards north Laos, Cambodia and finally Thailand, where we'd had the best, though still extortionate, quote to ship the truck to Australia.

Driving through Tibet was such a mix of the old and the new. There were traditional stone houses, but they were lit by brand-new solar-powered street lights and there was a ultra-modern highway on their doorstep. People were

Truck It!

labouring in the fields as they had done for centuries, but using Chinese-made tractors. There was a constant tension, which, once Sanghe had alluded to it, we couldn't unsee – a kind of quiet unhappiness.

One day there, we decided to stop and take a coach trip to Everest base camp on the northern side of the mountain. It is much higher than the Nepalese side, which is only accessible by a week's trekking.

'Ladies and gentlemen, over my shoulder, is Mount Everest!' was not a line I was ever expecting to be able to deliver to camera.

It was brutally cold, well below freezing when we visited, but incredibly dry. We got so close I swore if I focused hard enough, I would have been able to see any climbers if they had been summitting the highest mountain in the world. We took some snaps, videos and stood for as long as our fingers and toes could bear it.

I had read that there are over 200 unrecovered bodies currently on Everest. Eighteen people died there in 2023 alone. You know that with your head and yet, as I was staring up at it, you get that sense of why people want to climb it. It's just so enormous, so primal – what would it be like to stand on its summit?

'Don't even think about it,' said Marie, shaking her head as she saw something glinting in my eyes.

When we were back at the truck, the convoy of six vehicles agreed the next step with the guide, which was to get to a checkpoint two hours away. So, everyone jumped in their cars and vans and set off, but, as usual, we were scrambling to get packed up and the dogs in.

'Ah, crap,' I declared, after attempting, and failing, to bring the old girl to life. The fuel had frozen again.

'But we put minus-ten anti-freeze fuel in yesterday?' said Marie.

'Well, clearly not enough,' I said, letting out a big sigh, knowing some drama was about to play out.

I sent a message to the escort group, apologizing, as they were all already underway, and through complete luck managed to scavenge some wood from a building site next door, abandoned for the winter. Twenty minutes and one small careful fire later, now a self-declared professional fuel defroster, we were on our way. Elation from surviving yet another near miss was soon dampened by a fresh array of warning lights on the dashboard. So, once again under pressure from the convoy, we stopped during a lunch break to service the truck and replace all the fuel filters because the frozen fuel had dragged a load of crap through the fuel lines. It was freezing cold, and we were in the middle of nowhere on a Tibetan plateau, swearing, bodging, with frozen fingers – you get the picture by now. After three days of eight-hour drives, we reached the capital, Lhasa.

We had been told that Westerners would essentially be banned from travelling there, but we were allowed to walk around the city freely. It's an incredible place set in a valley in the Himalayas, and one of the highest cities in the world. We went to see Potala Palace, formerly the winter palace of the Dalai Lamas, which is an imposing building set into the red mountains, its ten-foot-thick walls supposedly containing a thousand rooms.

We also stopped off to see the seventh-century temple of

Truck It!

Jokhang, which is considered the spiritual heart of Tibetan Buddhism. The temple is a complex of different buildings surrounded by winding streets, and on one of these, thousands of people, young and old, walk around the temple for hours and hours, all wearing different outfits – from traditional Tibetan-style winter clothing to monks in simple shawls.

'Look at them,' said Marie, pointing towards a man and a boy, who had to be father and son.

They were covered in dirt, both wearing a leather apron and wooden blocks on each hand. They would take two steps forward, fall forwards onto the floor, then stand back up and pray. We watched and saw others doing the same movements. In front of the entrance, which had soft roll-up mats, they would do the same thing, but not moving forwards.

As we walked past one group, we heard a guide say, 'Keep an eye out for the devotees who pilgrimage to this holy site from every corner of Tibet. They do the prostrations all the way here.' It was a symbol of their commitment to their faith.

'That must have been that guy and his son,' I whispered to Marie, wondering how many hundred miles they had travelled like that. It put our grumbling about fuel freezing in perspective, that was for sure.

It was on our way east from Lhasa that we bashed mirrors with the Chinese Army. As I stood in the garage forecourt with a steadily more annoyed Chinese officer, I began to wonder if the next thing I was going to sightsee was the inside of a Chinese prison.

'You crash into truck. Commander very angry. You must pay or jail.'

'I'm terribly sorry but your driver crashed into me. Look,' waving the mirror guard in my hand. 'You must pay,' I said, holding my breath for a reaction.

His face flashed with shock and confusion.

He turned to his commander to translate and I thought, *Let's give it a go.*

So, I held the mirror guard high above my head, raised my voice and gave it the big guns: 'Who is going to pay for my truck? Your truck crashed into me. He was on my side of the road. This is very bad. My truck is very damaged. Cost a lot,' I said.

The translator gave it one last shot: 'You must pay.'

But I just carried on: 'You must pay for my truck, fella. This is very expensive. Yours is cheap. Mine very expensive. German. Who is paying me?'

Finally it was translated before the commander got bored and headed off to the comfort of his fake leather seats in his fake G-wagon.

'Try not to crash into anyone else,' said Marie with a smirk on her face as I tentatively climbed back into the cab. The soldiers were called back to the truck moments later and drove away.

Our fifteen days driving through China were incredibly varied, from the high Tibetan Plateau, which reminded me of Tajikistan in its harsh alien beauty, down through the mountains and then on into humid jungle. The one constant was the incredible food and the friendliness of the people we met. Oh, and the CCTV cameras. We left wanting to spend a year, or a decade, just exploring this enormous country, but

Truck It!

we knew that even a century would mean barely scratching the surface.

After 100 hours, and almost 2,000 miles of driving, carrying a broken motorbike on the truck's roof and dragging a broken-down car up and over 13,000ft passes, and coming to the aid of other members of the convoy as they encountered technical issues, we arrived at the border with Laos. We were elated, but utterly exhausted.

We'd made it to south-east Asia: Australia was now 'only' about 3,000 miles away.

25

Laos

'Bobby, quick!'

Marie's voice had a tone of panic I'd never heard before.

'It's Red. I . . . I think he's really hurt himself.'

I felt my stomach drop. We were halfway down a mountain we'd only just set off up, in the middle of a country I hadn't even heard of a month ago. It had been the only section of this mountain we could find that wasn't covered in completely impenetrable jungle, but it was still steep, slippery, and there were jagged rocks poking out beneath us.

We'd only got a hundred metres or so up when I realized things were getting a bit too hairy and that we were going to have to climb down or risk properly hurting ourselves. So that they didn't pull us off the ledge, we'd decided to set up a harness to get the dogs down, using a hammock to wrap

Truck It!

them up as they were lowered with a climbing rope. Once they were safe, Marie climbed down and I gathered all our stuff. And that's when I heard Marie's voice, hoarse with worry.

'Bobby! Oh god, there's blood everywhere.'

I took a deep breath and went to see what had happened.

It had felt like things had probably got a bit too relaxed. Two weeks earlier, we had crossed into the north of Laos from China without incident and had driven along winding roads through lush green hillsides covered in bamboo until we reached the town of Luang Prabang. It had once been famous for its traditional wooden houses, which look like the sails of a boat, but was now crowded with giftshops and tourists.

Early December in Laos is shorts and T-shirts weather, firmly at the beginning of the dry season, and Red and I hired a motorbike and did some exploring. After a couple of days of eating pizza and croissants, which were the things we'd missed the most as we'd crossed Asia, I started to get itchy feet. One night, I sat in the bar with a map.

'Right, I think it's time for another adventure. I'm sick of all this driving around,' I said. 'I think we should go paddleboarding and wild camping down the Mekong river.'

'You're crazy, you know that?' said Marie, taking a sip of her beer. 'What's on the Mekong river anyway?'

'It says here that, while it is synonymous with the role it played during the Vietnam conflict, the Mekong is one of the world's longest rivers and flows through one of the most biodiverse basins on the planet. We can paddle south for a few days, wild camping, until it intersects with the main highway maybe a hundred, a hundred and twenty-five kilometres away. Then I'm sure there will be some way of getting back.'

'Sounds good,' she said.

So, the following morning, having managed to locate and unpack all of our camping gear, we locked the truck, threw the kit and dogs onto the boards, and set off down the river. We left the town behind and soon were meandering our way through proper tropical jungle. Every now and then we would pass a tiny group of huts, and water buffalo wallowed at the water's edge as fishermen in wooden longboats cast their nets into the murky water. They stood and stared as two alien-looking foreigners with boards they had never seen before, overflowing with kit and dogs, drifted past. We would have to get more food at some point, but I figured if there were people, there was food, so we wouldn't starve.

'That'll do,' I pointed, half an hour before sunset. It was a small beach surrounded by jungle.

It had two trees leaning out over the river's edge, making it a perfect place to camp for the night.

We unloaded, built a little campfire, and hung the hammocks one on top of each other about three metres up the tree, then celebrated the sunset with two warm beers. I noticed again how much happier Marie was when we were in this kind of remote environment. She would make these little yelps of joy when she said something. And she rolled around with the dogs in the sand, laughing. It felt like for the first time since Afghanistan, she was able to unwind.

We kept our axe and knife within easy reach, but slept deeply, as we had our guard dogs beneath us on the floor, keeping out whatever was lurking inside the jungle on the edge of our camp. That first morning, we woke with the sunrise, swinging gently over the river, and I looked down at Marie, who had just woken up too. She looked so beautiful and so happy staring at the light on the water.

'What a life,' she whispered up to me, and I just nodded.

'I'm glad I went for that run,' she said.

'Me too,' I said, my voice catching.

And it was there I decided, who knows what would happen next, but I would try to make sure it had as many of these moments as humanly possible.

Over the next few days, we meandered down the Mekong river, living absolutely in the greatest moments of our lives. No distractions, simply watching rural Laos river life lazily slip past.

At one point, Marie went off into the jungle to see if she could find the owners of some fishing boats and buy some water. I sat waiting for twenty minutes, trying to ignore the worry that she had been kidnapped. Then I heard Rubia barking and stood up. Out of the jungle came Marie, followed by about twenty kids.

'You survived, then,' I said as she struggled her way down the beach with two big packs of bottled water.

'They were so lovely! We have noodles and water and they gave me this fizzy drink too!' she said, delighted.

After four long but beautiful days paddling down some of the wildest and most abstract landscapes we had seen so far, we were hungry and our arms were aching. As we looked out for somewhere suitable to camp in the fading light for our last night, it started to rain. To save on weight, we'd not packed the tent, figuring we'd camp under trees if it rained.

Now it was time to test that theory. Eventually we found a flat, muddy area, only just out of the waterline but sheltered by a thick canopy overhead. We landed the paddleboards, offloaded, and began chopping our way through vines, old bamboo shoots and ant nests to make some space to sleep. We were ankle deep in mud as we flipped a paddleboard and made a walkway of tree branches to attempt to keep us dry as we ate the last of our supplies, huddled by the fire. We played cards under torchlight.

'Life can't all be sunrises,' I said. 'If it were all lottery wins, sunrises and long lunches, you wouldn't appreciate it. I'll take some hard graft and testing moments to keep me feeling alive.'

'Well, this isn't so bad,' said Marie, playing the winning hand for the sixth time straight.

The following day, we came to a bridge over the river flanked by rural villages. As we were negotiating a price back to Luang Prabang, villagers arrived with a wild boar on a boat and proceeded to sell bits of it to the highest bidders. Our chariot was a barely drivable people-carrier that bounced us the four hours as the crow flies back north. But that evening, as we were just starting to think about leaving for Cambodia, Marie was flicking through her passport when she suddenly stopped.

'*Merde!*' she exclaimed, throwing her passport down.

'What's the matter, Baguette?'

'I don't have room for any more stamps. They won't let me in without a stamp.'

'Well, we'd better sort another passport, then,' I said.

Three days later, after a call with the embassy, I dropped

Truck It!

Marie at Vang Vieng to catch a Chinese-built bullet train to the capital, Vientiane. We had been warned that her new passport could take anything up to five weeks to arrive, which was three more weeks than we'd planned on staying. But we decided that was a tomorrow problem, and when she arrived back, I suggested we go and camp in the mountains.

And that's when I heard the tone of worry in her voice I had never heard before.

'Bobby, quickly!'

I climbed back up the steep cliff far too quickly until I was just below them. Red was standing very still and I could see his fur matted with blood, but his tail was wagging and he still had a big smile on his face with his tongue hanging out. I climbed as far as I was able to get, then whistled for him to come down to me. It was too dangerous for me to get to where they were, but unless things were very bad, he should be able to get down to me. He looked like he was walking pretty normally, jumping down a couple of little steps, before arriving level with my head for the last big jump. I caught him around the stomach, and immediately knew we were all in trouble. My fingers were touching something wet and warm and it felt like I was holding raw chicken breast. I swung him round and placed him gently down on the wooden platform. I pulled my hand from under his belly and my right hand was covered in blood.

'Ah, mate, come here. Are you alright?' I said to Red, who was looking back up at Rubia and Marie, who were climbing down to get to us.

I knelt down and saw a hole in his stomach about six inches wide and the same long.

'He jumped down to that flat ledge but there was a tiny rock sticking out and he snagged his belly on it,' said Marie.

'Okay, let me take a look.' I grabbed him, and gently flipped him on his side.

'Alright, this isn't going to be nice, but needs doing straight away,' I said pulling out a two-litre bottle of water.

I cracked the lid and began gently washing out the wound. Red lay obediently without moving a muscle or making a noise. I felt incredible sorry and proud of my little soldier for being such a tough cookie.

I washed the wound of little stones and vegetation, then wrapped him in Marie's T-shirt before we lifted him up to start the walk back to the truck, which must have been nearly ten kilometres away.

'Honestly, he doesn't want to be carried,' I said as we stood two minutes later. He normally accepted being carried, but was putting up a bit of a fight.

'Maybe it's putting pressure on the wound?' said Marie.

'Are you sure, mate?' I said, looking at Red, who was looking back at me wagging his tail. 'Alright, come on then, you tough bastard.'

For over an hour, Red walked off lead to heel, with a hole the size of a plate in his stomach, until we reached the truck.

'It says here there's a vet,' said Marie, furiously scrolling on her phone as I drove much too fast back towards the nearest town. 'Forty-five minutes away.'

Up until that moment, I had been trying to work out a contingency plan for no vet, which included sewing him up myself, or supergluing the wound shut, which we had successfully done when he was a puppy when we had a less dramatic but similar incident in Scotland in the middle of nowhere.

'I'm sorry I got you into this, mate,' I said, looking at him.

When we got to the 'vet', it turned out to be a run-down store with shelves of cokes, ice creams, pot noodles and some dog and cat food.

'I'm not sure this is a vet,' I said as I jumped out.

An old guy wearing a grubby football shirt, tracksuit bottoms and flip-flops came out and looked at me with curiosity.

I tried to explain that Red needed stitching up and asked if he could help. He beckoned for me to bring Red and follow him into the back. I don't know what I was expecting, but the back was a shed attached to the open-fronted dusty store. It was, and this is saying something, even dirtier than the truck. But there was a stainless steel table that didn't look too bad, so I popped my little fella on it. Without saying a word to Red or us, he gave him a quick once-over, playing with his wound with unwashed hands, before disappearing off. A minute later, he reappeared and, again silently, injected him. My heart sank to what felt like my feet.

'Sleep,' he said, and went off to serve someone in the shop. I watched as the unknown, unmeasured jab took effect and Red's head began to drop.

Once his eyes began to slowly shut, the realization that he might never wake up overwhelmed me. The guy hadn't weighed him, or checked him. Who knows what he'd just injected into him. I had my head against his, whispering and crying into his fur as he fought to stay awake.

'You're my best mate, Red. I love you so much. I wouldn't have got through these past couple of years without you. Thank you for being my best mate. I love you, mate. I'm so sorry.'

I was suddenly dizzy and started to stumble. Marie sprung over to me and put her arms under my armpits as I grabbed the table. The guy came back in and I didn't know whether to punch him or plead with him.

'Please,' I said. 'Please help him.'

He stroked Red's face, then set about shaving the hair from around the cut with a loose razor blade, before grabbing medieval-looking instruments and sewing him up.

Halfway through, he stopped, shouted something to a woman who appeared grumpily in pyjamas holding a pair of glasses. He put them on and turned to me.

'Can't see,' he laughed.

The sight of the fur, blood and Red twisting and turning every so often as this ill-kept butcher sewed him up was too much. Marie quickly dragged a chair over and pushed it behind my knees as I collapsed down onto it.

I'd seen my share of broken bones on the rugby field, including a bone sticking out of my own finger, a four-inch hole in my own head, and once my mum had broken her ankle so badly her foot was pointing the wrong way, but this was worse than that.

Fifteen stressful minutes later, he proudly announced 'Done,' dropping the bloody instruments and inspecting his work.

A long, jagged set of stitches ran across his shaved belly, angry and red, the skin bulging around the wound.

Truck It!

'Come on, mate,' I said. 'Wake up.'

I sat there for half an hour, stroking his head and whispering to him before I saw his tongue start to move. Then his eyes struggled open and he lifted his head up. He was confused and dopey, but he was awake.

'Let's get out of here, mate,' I whispered as I scooped him up and carried him back to the truck, abandoned on the street outside.

'Forty dollars,' the 'vet' said as I went back to pay, still wiping blood from his hands with an old rag, and Red's blood splattered all down his football shirt.

Red was still unsteady on his feet, so we found a quiet spot to park and I sat with him, stroking his head. It took me a few hours to let him out of my sight at all. And for days afterwards, I'd get worried if I couldn't find him immediately.

After all that drama, we dialled down the adventure for the next couple of weeks. We still spent Christmas Eve in a cave and exploring the local countryside on what is known as the Thakhek Loop, parking up next to deserted rivers, swimming and drinking the very reasonable local beer, which was cheaper than water. Then we wound our way down towards Pakse to see the new year in. The south of the country was incredible, and every night we found a new spot near a river or waterfall where we were the only humans for miles.

As I danced with Marie on New Year's Eve to a dodgy Queen tribute band, I thought how far we'd come. Thirty-four countries and over 30,000 miles driven. We'd swum in at least a couple of hundred lakes and rivers, and seen a few hundred sunsets and sunrises. We'd eaten incredible food (some of which had stayed down), and we'd seen the absolute best of what humanity had to offer. Kindness and generosity beyond anything I could imagine.

And I'd got engaged to the funniest, most joyful person I'd ever known. I'd gone from someone who couldn't imagine a future where I was happy, to being grateful every day for the gift of life. And, to cap it off, we were within touching distance of our goal. Australia was somewhere out beyond that horizon waiting for us.

If the next year was even half as good as the previous one, I couldn't wait.

Epilogue

'Well, that's it, then,' I said. 'We're officially effed.'

I sat looking at the email from Australia's Department for Fisheries and Forestry. It said that, before we could enter the country, Red and Rubia would need to be quarantined for six months. And not in the same place we'd be shipping the truck to.

I texted Marie, who was 200 miles north of me, still in Laos. We had temporarily parted ways after an amazing few weeks exploring Don Det and other islands in the middle of the Mekong in the south of the country, swimming, eating and watching the sun rise and set over the wooden guest-houses that dotted the riverbanks.

I was about to head further south into Cambodia with the truck and the dogs, so that she could wait for her new passport to arrive and I could write the book that you're now reading, so we wanted to spend some proper time all together. We also knew that there was going to be the complication of getting the truck and then the dogs into Australia.

We were aware that the fact that we'd been through so many countries without any official vet documentation for the dogs meant that we could fall foul of the most extreme quarantine laws, but had sent off an optimistic email.

I hugged Marie for a long time in the parking area next to the truck. This three weeks would be the longest we'd been apart since we'd met.

'I love you,' I whispered.

'Je t'aime,' Marie whispered back as we kissed goodbye and she made a final fuss of the dogs.

Then, I had set off south, negotiating my way out of spending about a hundred dollars to pay the ten bribes at the border into Cambodia, pausing only to get stuck in a car park, which the local old boys found extremely funny, until, during the rescue attempts, I crashed the truck into a wall.

I spent long days editing the diary I'd been keeping wherever possible, and fleshing it out into the sort of story that resembled something actually readable (and I guess that must have worked if you have stuck with it this far!).

I'd just pressed send to my editor, sat back and cracked open a beer, when the email from the Australian Fisheries and Forestry department arrived.

I took the dogs for a walk as I tried to work out what to do. Shipping the truck to Australia would absolutely clean us out, and there was no way we could afford to wait while the dogs spent all that time on their own. Six bloody months! What a joke!

On the phone that evening, Marie suggested her mum could look after them for a couple of months if we could somehow get them back to France, and then the two of us could carry on the journey without them.

'But, Marie, it's *all of our* journey. Both of them too,' I said.

After a rocky start with Rubia, I had grown to love her – as had Red. The thought of crossing the finish line without them felt like no finish at all.

'Well, okay then, James Bond. What's the grand plan?'

I genuinely didn't know. All I knew was that we needed to be together and there was no way I was done. There had to be some kind of solution.

The next day, I got a text from Marie out of the blue.

'Didn't you tell me this is all about the journey and not the destination?'

'Yeah, so?'

'You'll figure it out.'

That night, inspiration hit me, and I put in a call to the Thai shipping company.

Eureka.

The next day, I drove to meet Marie in Phnom Penh. As the dogs and I sat patiently in front of the truck, Marie sneaked up and surprised the two furballs, who went bananas.

'Well?' she said.

'I might have an idea,' I said. 'But first we need to get into Thailand.'

'What's the plan?' she said.

'Well, I need to turn the blag up to eleven for this one.

No trucks, campervans or any foreign vehicle over three and a half tonnes can enter.'

'So, we're breaking all three rules in one go, then?'

'Correct,' I said matter-of-factly. 'So, the plan is to try to sneak into Thailand, then blag it. I've got the shipping info printed, a fake hotel booking, ours and the dogs' flights home, the old set of car import permit rules . . .'

Five days later, we stood with big puppy-dog eyes, looking directly into the whites of the eyes of the head of customs for the Thai border.

'Sir, it is completely not permitted. I'm sorry but you are going to have to turn back.'

'But if you would just give me a second to explain . . .'

'Sir, please, you are blocking traffic. You must go back.'

Marie, not for the first time on the trip, was blissfully chatting to someone on the far side of the border, having been stamped into Thailand without drama.

With a handful of paperwork and a sorry look on my face, I waved, caught her eye and shook my head.

'Why?' I just about heard over the noise of the busy border, as trucks, people and cars weaved their way through all the checkpoints.

'For god's sake,' I said, getting back into the truck, throwing the paperwork onto the dashboard as the dogs looked innocently back to check I was okay. I had a plan B, but even that needed us to be in Thailand. I put my head on the dashboard and closed my eyes. That was that. We'd have to admit defeat. I'd have to admit to Marie that I'd mucked it up. I'd have to admit to the *world* that I'd mucked up. Unless . . .

Truck It!

As the paperwork spread down the dash, I saw a printout of our shipping booking.

I never thought I'd be grateful to the Taliban, but in that moment, I had a sudden flash of memory – of the feeling of terror when he'd picked up the phone and called the number. *One last go, Bobby.*

Somehow, I managed to convince the friendliest customs officer to call our shipping agent in Thailand, who wasn't expecting a call.

All I can say is, he must have been brought up being taught the same valuable life lessons in blagging as myself.

'Yes, it's essential they are allowed through. The ship is waiting for them. They plan on driving straight to the port and loading this evening,' he said in perfect Thai.

He really turned it on. All the way up to eleven. An eight out of ten probably would have worked, but as the chief of customs fudged our import permit to allow us to cross, I really wouldn't have cared if I'd had to take it up another notch and called myself Billy.

So, by the skin of our teeth, we made it into Thailand. With one last call to the shipping company to confirm the arrangements, we drove to a deserted beach in time for sunset.

I opened a bottle of warm champagne and went to join Marie.

'Happy Birthday to you,' I sang.

She swigged from the bottle. 'Well, is it official?'

'It is,' I said.

'Tomorrow, we ship the truck to South Africa!' she laughed and clapped her hands. 'I'd better tell my mum!'

This was my new plan: we would fly to Cape Town, join the truck, and then begin the 7,000-mile drive up the length of Africa, back up to Europe.

'To the journey,' she said.

'To the journey,' I agreed. I put my arm around her and we watched the sun set as the dogs ran on the beach.

For the final time, that night, while Marie toasted a marshmallow over the fire with the dogs lying snoozing on the beach, I pulled out my diary for the final time.

Well that's a wrap . . . or is it?

Australia was the chequered flag, luring me to the far side of the world, but driving to within touching distance turned out to be a springboard, maybe even a life-raft my life so desperately needed.

What played out I could not have hoped, nor dreamt, nor paid enough for.

It has been wilder, crazier, worse and more beautiful than any story I've ever read.

Not making OZ is as much of a thing to celebrate as it is a disappointment.

Because not making Australia proves the end has not been reached.

No.

This is just the beginning.

I closed my journal, picked up a stick, loaded on a marshmallow and looked over at the love of my life, lost in her own thoughts, staring into the flames dancing out from the fire.

I decided to save the fact that the truck didn't fit in the shipping container for another time.

That was tomorrow's problem.

Acknowledgements

I can remember our first chat with Lydia Ramah from Pan Macmillan who asked if we would consider writing a book about our journey. Rather fittingly, we were pulled over on a precarious mountain pass, over 13,000ft above sea level in central Asia, and the incoming snow blizzard was disrupting our signal. I don't think we both knew what we were getting ourselves into, but I'm incredibly grateful for the opportunity to share our story.

So, thank you to Lydia and the rest of the team of Victoria Denne and Meg Le Huquet, for their continued support and quick adaptability in helping to pull this off, while we continued to travel around the world. This book was written around the world, partially drafted in Pakistan, typed up in Cambodia, edited while swinging in a hammock on a Thai island, checked on a plane back to Europe and signed off in the cab of our next adventure truck while in England.

Special thanks must go to our editor, Jamie Coleman, who,

and I'm still not sure how, was able to transform the ramblings of a madman who should have paid more attention in English at school, into a fast-paced, punchy book of which I am incredibly proud. His job title should be 'Magician', not 'Editor'.

To my mum, my dad, Stephen, Karen and my grandparents, I want to say thank you for putting up with me over the years and for giving me a nice hard shove in the right direction when required. I simply would not be the same guy had you not inspired me with your strong work ethic and persistent drive towards success. I fear I will never truly be able to pay you back for your support.

And finally, thank you to Marie for following her heart and rolling the dice on date three. This story, journey or new chapter in my life would be nowhere near as fulfilling had fate not brought us together for sunrise on the top of that mountain. I can't wait to call you my wife.